Jamie H Schneider

Instruction
SUGGESTED LIST PR...

TIMES MIRROR

THE C. V. MOSBY COMPANY
11830 WESTLINE INDUSTRIAL DRIVE
ST. LOUIS, MISSOURI 63141

COMPREHENSIVE REVIEW
FOR MEDICAL TECHNOLOGISTS

MOSBY'S COMPREHENSIVE REVIEW SERIES

Comprehensive review for medical technologists

EDITED BY

Alice M. Semrad

Director of Medical Technology,
Marquette University,
Milwaukee, Wisconsin

THE C. V. MOSBY COMPANY

SAINT LOUIS   1975

Library of Congress Cataloging in Publication Data

Semrad, Alice M   1929-
  Comprehensive review for medical technologists.

  (Mosby's comprehensive review series)
  Includes index.
  1. Medicine, Clinical—Outlines, syllabi, etc.
I. Title. [DNLM: 1. Technology, Medical. QY25 S473c]
RB37.S45   616'.002'02   74-28379
ISBN 0-8016-4486-0

VH/VH/VH   9 8 7 6 5 4 3 2 1

Contributors

■ **Edwin L. Bemis, M.D., F.C.A.P., F.A.S.C.P.**
Associate Director of Laboratories and Vice Chief of Medical Staff, Deaconess Hospital; Assistant Clinical Professor of Pathology, Medical College of Wisconsin; Lecturer in Medical Technology, Marquette University, Milwaukee, Wisconsin

■ **Anthony Cafaro, M.D., F.C.A.P., F.A.S.C.P.**
Associate Pathologist, St. Joseph's Hospital; Lecturer in Medical Technology, Marquette University, Milwaukee, Wisconsin

■ **Silas G. Farmer, Ph.D.**
Microbiologist, Milwaukee County Medical Complex; Associate Professor of Pathology, Medical College of Wisconsin; Clinical Professor of Microbiology, Marquette University School of Dentistry; Fellow, American Academy of Microbiology; Diplomate, American Board of Medical Microbiology; Lecturer in Medical Technology, Marquette University, Milwaukee, Wisconsin

■ **Opal Kelly, M.T. (ASCP)**
Medical Technologist Supervisor, Milwaukee County Medical Complex; Lecturer in Medical Technology, Marquette University, Milwaukee, Wisconsin

■ **Gordon Lang, M.D., F.C.A.P., F.A.S.C.P.**
Associate Pathologist, St. Mary's Hospital; Lecturer in Medical Technology, Marquette University, Milwaukee, Wisconsin

■ **Alfred Meyers, M.D., F.C.A.P., F.A.S.C.P.**
Associate Pathologist, St. Mary's Hospital; Assistant Clinical Professor in Pathology, Medical College of Wisconsin; Lecturer in Medical Technology, Marquette University, Milwaukee, Wisconsin

■ **John D. Reeves, M.S., M.T. (ASCP)**

Instructor in Medical Technology, Marquette University, Milwaukee, Wisconsin

■ **Joan Shrout, B.S., M.T. (ASCP)**

Clinical Instructor in Medical Technology, Marquette University; Clinical Instructor in Chemistry, St. Mary's Hospital, Milwaukee, Wisconsin

■ **Raymond Zastrow, M.Ed., M.D., F.C.A.P.**

Pathologist and Director of Radio Chemistry, St. Michael's Hospital; Assistant Clinical Professor of Pathology, Medical College of Wisconsin; Lecturer in Medical Technology, Marquette University, Milwaukee, Wisconsin; Member, American College of Nuclear Physicians

Preface

Upon arriving at the close of academic preparation for a career as a medical laboratory technologist, a student will have reached a career milestone. College and clinical education (internship) are designed to prepare each student to be a competent technologist. The next goal is certification or licensure. This book was written to help the reader review the academic background so that this goal can be achieved successfully.

This book is intended only as a review mechanism. It does not provide detailed explanations. Students should consider the questions contained herein, determine whether or not they understand the concepts and facts presented, and from this return to their textbooks and personal notes for further study as needed.

The authors have not dealt with methodology but rather with the understanding of laboratory procedures and all their ramifications. The student should not memorize such details of procedures as amounts of reagents used but rather should concentrate on their sequence in the procedure and the reason for their use. To help the student review, we have included outlines that may be used as study guides. Also included is a listing of procedures that the student should have studied throughout the year of clinical work. This listing represents the type of procedures one would find available to the physicians on the staff of a modern, average-sized, urban hospital, short of the status of a research center. By referring to the list of procedures and asking the questions contained in the appropriate outlines, the student should have an organized method of review.

The education of medical laboratory technologists extends beyond that of medical laboratory technicians so that they may not only perform laboratory procedures but also be able to correlate, interpret, compare, and analyze them. The questions in this book were devised to assist in achieving this objective.

The student should not be apprehensive regarding the mechanics and the format of the examination. The examination of the Board of Registry of the American Society of Clinical Pathology contains 200 items of the multiple-choice type. Only one answer is considered correct and this answer is marked on the standard answer sheet to be scored by a computer. Frequently there is more than one possible answer. Since the best choice is the most correct answer, the examinee should be careful to analyze all choices before selecting the final answer.

Examinees who feel great anxiety over the examination should purchase a handbook on how to take an examination. These are available in most college or university bookstores. The education coordinator who sent the approval to the Board of Registry verifying an individual's eligibility to take the examination did so with the conviction that the applicant would successfully pass the examination. Achieving a passing score on an examination that leads to successful certification or licensure is only part of the medical technologist's goal. Technical competence must accompany successful certification or licensure for those who wish to practice as professional medical laboratory technologists. It is appropriate to begin this review with an honest self-assessment of one's technical competence. The review should be started 6 weeks before an examination is to be taken. Those having doubts regarding their technical competence should return to their practicum teachers in the laboratory to review techniques. Without technical competence, academic competence is of little value in the laboratory.

Because of the rising trend to make continuing education a contingency for continued certification and licensure, the authors hope that this book will serve as a source of reference for persons seeking insight into current theories and practices in the medical laboratory. In addition to senior medical technology students, the following individuals will also find this book helpful: (1) practicing technologists who wish to update their information either in the area of medical technology in which they are currently engaged, or in an area to which they wish to transfer their interest, (2) technologists wishing to return to work after a number of years of absence from the laboratory, (3) persons wishing to prepare for academic equivalency examinations given by the College-Level Examination Program (CLEP) of the College Examination Board, Princeton, New Jersey.

This book is the result of the cooperative effort of many. They have attempted to give the student or examinee a concise guide for study. We are indebted to the student readers, Holly Frisby, Mary Jo Steele, and Barbara Tomcko, and the student indexer, Ann Grotelueschen. We are further grateful to Mrs. Katherine Christensen for her assistance in coordinating the text, and to Miss Kaye Cullen for the listing of laboratory tests.

ALICE M. SEMRAD

Study guide for students

CLINICAL MICROBIOLOGY

A. Name and classification of infectious agent
B. Methodology
   1. Collection and handling of specimen
      a. Source of specimen
      b. Aseptic technique required
   2. Identification
      a. Cellular morphology and staining
      b. Colonial characteristics
      c. Growth requirements
         (1) Nutritional (known media components and the reason for their use)
            (a) For isolation
            (b) For differentiation
         (2) Atmospheric
   3. Serologic reactions
   4. Antibiotic susceptibility
C. Pathogenicity
   1. Pathologic process resulting from infection
      a. Relationship of process to laboratory findings (serology, hematology, chemistry)
      b. Immunologic response
   2. Transmission
   3. Epidemiology

CLINICAL CHEMISTRY

A. Name of substance to be analyzed
   1. Chemical classification of compound
   2. Reference method
   3. Routine chemical method
B. Methodology
   1. Outline the procedure step by step, including:
      a. How to obtain the specimen
      b. How to preserve the specimen

2. Discuss the chemistry of the procedure, i.e., the purpose of each step and chemistry involved (when a particular instrument is used discuss it and its application)
3. Sources of errors in the procedure (endogenous and exogenous)
4. Quality control
5. Quality assurance
6. Contraindications in using the procedure
7. Advantages and disadvantages of the procedure

C. Pathophysiology
1. The normal physiologic and biochemical relationships of the substance with related anatomy
2. Conditions in the patient resulting in variations in the physiology and biochemistry leading to abnormal values (high or low)
3. Relationship of this substance to other laboratory findings

CLINICAL MICROSCOPY*

A. Choice of type of microscopy and light source
B. Preparation of the material to be viewed
C. Characteristics to be examined:
1. Size
2. Shape
3. Symmetry
4. Thickness (e.g., third dimension or depth of form)
5. Consistency (e.g., light transmission)
6. Constituents or components (e.g., structural units)
7. Movement (if any)

PROCEDURES FOR CHEMISTRY

Acid phosphatase	Blood gases and electrolytes
Albumin	pH
Albumin binding capacity	P_{CO_2}
Alcohol level	P_{O_2}
Alkaline phosphatase	P50
Ammonia	CO
Amylase	CO_2
Barbiturate level	% Oxygen saturation
Bilirubin	Osmolality measurement

*This outline can be used whether it be the microscopic study of urinary sediment, blood smears for hematologic studies, or microbiologic studies.

Chloride
Lithium
Potassium
Sodium
BSP
BUN
Calcium
Cholesterol
CPK
Creatinine
Creatinine clearance
Diagnex blue
2,3-DPG
Gamma glutamyl transfers
  (GGT)
Gastric analysis
Glucose
Hemoglobin

Iron-binding capacity
Iron serum
Lactate levels
LDH
Lipase
Lipids (total)
Magnesium
5′ Nucleotidase
Phosphorus (inorganic)
Protein (total)
PSP
Salicylate level
Serotonin
SGOT
SGPT
Stone analysis
Triglyceride
Uric acid

PROCEDURES FOR COAGULATION

Circulating anticoagulant tests
Clot retraction
Correction of abnormal pro-
  thrombin time
Duke bleeding time
Euglobulin clot lysis
Factor assay (intrinsic and ex-
  trinsic)
Fibrin split products
Fibrin stabilizing factor, 5M
  urea test for
Fibrinogen assay
Heparin neutralization
Ivy bleeding time
Lee-White whole blood clotting
  time

Make-up corrective plasmas
  and serum
Partial thromboplastin time
Plasma recalcification time
Platelet screening
Protamine paracoagulation
Prothrombin consumption
  time
Prothrombin time
Reptilase time
Rumple-Leeds test
Stypven time
Thrombin time
Thromboplastin generation
  time

PROCEDURES FOR HEMATOLOGY

Autohemolysin test
Bone marrow prep

Cytogenetics
Culture

Karyotyping
Differential counts—peripheral and bone marrow
Electrophoresis—hemoglobin, haptoglobin
Fragility tests—osmotic, mechanical, acid
Giemsa stain
G_6PDH—assay, fluorescent, ascorbate-cyanide
Heinz body stain
Hematocrit
Hemoglobin
Histiocyte smear
Indices calculation
Kliehauer stain
LE—standard, fluorescent
Leukocyte alkaline phosphatase stain

Malaria smears (thick and thin)
Mechanical fragility
Nasal smear for eosinophils
Nitroblue tetrazolium stain
Osmotic fragility
Particle counts
   Automated
   Manual (WBC, RBC, platelets, eosinophils, and sperm)
Periodic acid–Schiff stain
Peroxidase stain
Reticulocyte count
Sedimentation rate
Sickle cell preparation
Sickledex
Spinal fluid cell count
Sudan black B stain
Wright's stain

PROCEDURES FOR IMMUNOHEMATOLOGY

ABO typing
ABO typing discrepancies
Absorption elution
Amniocentesis
Antenatal workup
Antibody screening
Antigen typing and identification
Component therapy
Coombs testing
Cord blood studies
Crossmatch
Du testing

Family studies
Genotyping
Hemolysis A and B
Identification panel
Immune A and B titer
Incompatible crossmatch
Leukagglutinins
Rh titration
Rh typing
RhoGam procedure
Subgrouping
Transfusion reaction

PROCEDURES FOR SEROLOGY

Alpha antitrypsin
Alpha fetoglobin
Amebiasis
Antihyaluronidase

ASO titer
C reactive protein
Cold agglutinins
Complement levels

Erythropoietin levels
Febrile agglutination
Fibrin split products
Hemagglutination inhibition
Histoplasmosis
Leptospirosis
Migratory inhibition factor
Monospot
Neuramidase

Rheumatoid arthritis
RPR
Rubella
T cells
Thyroid antibody test
Toxoplasmosis
Trichinosis
VDRL

INFECTIOUS AGENTS FOR MICROBIOLOGY*

Micrococcus
Staphylococcus
Gaffkya
Streptococcus
Enterococcus (Streptococcus faecalis)
Pneumococcus (Streptococcus pneumoniae)
Neisseria
Pseudomonas
Moraxella
Actinobacter
Flavobacterium
Xanthomonas
Alcaligenes
Escherichia
Shigella
Edwardsiella
Salmonella
Arizona
Citrobacter
Klebsiella
Enterobacter
Serratia
Proteus
Yersinia
Vibrio
Haemophilus

Bordetella
Brucella
Pasteurella
Francisella
Bacillus
Corynebacterium
Listeria
Erysipelothrix
Clostridium
Bifidobacterium
Propionibacterium
Eubacterium
Lactobacillus
Actinomyces
Arachnia
Bacteroides
Fusobacterium
Peptococcus
Peptostreptococcus
Veillonella
Mycobacterium
Spirillum
Borrelia
Treponema
Leptospira
Aeromonas
Streptobacillus
Mycoplasma

*Identify the clinically significant species of the following genera.

INFECTIOUS AGENTS FOR PARASITOLOGY*

Cestodes
  Diphyllobothrium latum
  Dipylidium caninum
  Echinococcus granulosus
  Echinococcus multilocularis
  Hymenolepis diminuta
  Hymenolepis nana
  Taenia saginata
  Taenia solium
Nematodes
  Acanthocheilonema perstans
  Ancylostoma braziliense
  Ancylostoma duodenale
  Ascaris lumbricoides
  Enterobius vermicularis
  Loa loa
  Mansonella ozzardi
  Necator americanus
  Onchocerca volvulus
  Strongyloides stercoralis
  Toxocara canis
  Toxocara cati
  Trichinella spiralis
  Trichuris trichiura
  Wuchereria bancrofti
  Wuchereria malayi
Protozoa
  Balantidium coli
  Chilomastix mesnili
  Dientamoeba fragilis

Endolimax nana
Entamoeba coli
Entamoeba gingivalis
Entamoeba histolytica
Giardia lamblia
Iodamoeba buetschlii
Leishmania braziliensis
Leishmania donovani
Leishmania tropica
Plasmodium falciparum
Plasmodium malariae
Plasmodium ovale
Plasmodium vivax
Toxoplasma gondii
Trichomonas hominis
Trichomonas tenax
Trichomonas vaginalis
Trypanosoma cruzi
Trypanosoma gambiense
Trypanosoma rhodesiense
Trematodes
  Clonorchis sinensis
  Fasciola hepatica
  Fasciolopsis buski
  Heterophyes heterophyes
  Paragonimus westermani
  Schistosoma dermatitis
  Schistosoma haematobium
  Schistosoma japonicum
  Schistosoma mansoni

PROCEDURES FOR URINALYSIS

Physical properties
  Physical appearance
  Specific gravity
Chemical properties
  Bilirubin

Glucose
Ketones
Occult blood
pH
Protein

---

*Identify the clinically significant stages.

Addis count

Aminoacidurias

Bence Jones protein

Calcium

Concentration and dilution
   tests

Crystal identification

Hemosiderin

Homogentisic acid

Human chorionic gonadotropin

Melanin

Porphobilinogen

PROCEDURES FOR STOOL ANALYSIS

Fat

Meat fibers

Occult blood

Starch

Trypsin

Contents

CHAPTER 1

Hemostasis

EDWIN L. BEMIS

■ **What is a convenient classification of hemorrhagic disorders?**

There are two main types of hemorrhagic disease: primary disorders, which are usually congenital; and secondary disorders, which are acquired and are related to some other underlying disease. Whether primary or secondary, they may be most conveniently classified as dependent upon the defect of the supportive tissues about blood vessels, of the blood vessels themselves, of blood platelets, or of blood plasma.

■ **What are some examples of extravascular (tissue) bleeding disorders?**

The Ehlers-Danlos syndrome is a hereditary form of bleeding disorder associated with marked hyperelasticity and fragility of the skin. Acquired abnormalities include "senile purpura" associated with degenerative changes of supportive tissues, and "post-menopausal purpura," which is as yet poorly understood.

■ **What are some examples of vascular bleeding disorders?**

Perhaps the most obvious example of vascular bleeding disorder is injury that causes loss of integrity of blood vessels, allowing blood to leak out. The hereditary vascular abnormalities include hereditary telangiectasia and the Minot-von Willebrand syndrome ("pseudohemophilia"). Hereditary telangiectasia is extremely uncommon and consists of tiny dilatations of capillaries and venules in the skin and mucous membranes particularly. The Minot-von Willebrand syndrome is the most common hereditary hemorrhagic disease known. It is transmitted as an autosomal dominant and therefore appears in both males and females with approximately equal incidence. The true defect is unknown but

1

many believe it to be associated with a decreased "antibleeding" substance, which is necessary to maintain vascular ingregity. Acquired disorders in which vascular damage is the major cause of bleeding include syphilis and arteriosclerosis, in which rupture of an aneurysm is the common hemorrhagic manifestation. "Acquired vascular purpura" is a term used to indicate that hemorrhagic manifestations are directly related to vascular damage. This may be associated with a wide variety of agents that increase the permeability of vessel lining (endothelial cells), resulting in petechiae and purpura. Such disorders include: damage from immunologic reactions, termed "allergic vasculitis," of which Schoenlein-Henoch purpura is one type; those that may also be associated with obstruction of vessels such as sometimes occurs when there are abnormal proteins (e.g., cryoglobulins) or bacteria (e.g., meningococci) in the blood; and vitamin C deficiency (scurvy), because this vitamin is required to maintain the cement substance (hyaluronic acid) between endothelial cells.

■ **What laboratory test abnormalities may be expected in patients with the Minot-von Willebrand syndrome?**

The one most characteristic test abnormality is a prolonged bleeding time. However, this may be normal but platelet adhesiveness will be abnormal. Most investigators also require demonstration of decreased antihemophilic globulin (factor VIII) for the diagnosis. The Rumpel-Leede test may also be positive.

■ **Are hereditary disorders of platelets common?**

No, they are rare. Most of the primary quantitative defects of platelets have been associated with decreased numbers of megakaryocytes in the bone marrow. The hereditary, functional, or qualitative platelet disorders include Glanzmann's thrombasthenia associated with defective glycolysis of platelets and markedly abnormal clot retraction; and congenital thrombopathia, in which there is defective release of phospholipids from platelets.

■ **What is the most common cause of hemorrhagic disease?**

An acquired disorder of platelets is the most common cause of hemorrhagic disease. Decreased numbers of platelets may result from decreased platelet production or from increased removal of platelets from the circulation. Common causes of decreased platelet production are diseases in which the number of megakaryocytes in the bone marrow is reduced. Typical examples include "aplastic" anemia and conditions associated with replacement of the bone marrow by tumor cells (as in leukemia) or by inflammatory tissue. Increased rate of removal of platelets from the circulation may be caused by the presence of antiplatelet factors ("immunologic thrombocytopenia"), such as may develop following the administration of certain drugs, after blood transfusions, in newborn infants, following viral infection, or occurring for reasons unknown (idiopathically). Thrombocytopenia is also seen on occasion following a single massive thrombosis or in association with innumerable tiny clotted vessels. Following hemorrhage and massive replacement with stored (platelet-poor) blood, thrombocytopenia may result from simple dilution. Certain diseases of "platelet sequestering areas," particularly the spleen, probably also represent examples of increased removal of platelets from the circulating blood. Acquired, functional disorders of platelets are associated with deficient synthesis of phospholipids by platelets and are occasionally seen in association with such disorders as uremia, leukemia, liver disease, and polycythemia vera.

■ **What are the clinical and laboratory characteristics of bleeding caused by platelet abnormalities?**

As with disorders involving blood vessels, platelet abnormalities may be characterized by surface bleeding such as petechiae or purpura along with nasal, gastrointestinal, or intrauterine bleeding. Laboratory characteristics of this group include a prolonged bleeding time with variable alteration of the tourniquet test and of tests for the first stage of coagulation (which may be corrected by the addition of platelets or a platelet substitute such as cephaloplastin or hemolyzed red blood cells). Separate tests of platelet function include those for platelet adhesiveness and platelet aggregation. Rarely, only prolongation of the bleeding time may be present with no other demonstrable abnormality; this is referred to as "athrombia." Here it is postulated that the agglutinating ability of platelets is impaired and that they cannot undergo orderly viscous metamorphosis.

■ **What is "primary hemostasis?"**

When a small blood vessel is cut, a series of events occurs, the first two simultaneously: contraction of the vessel wall and disruption of the endothelial lining with exposure of the collagen layer to the lumen. Platelets are then adsorbed on the collagen and liberate many components including serotonin, which further enhances vascular constriction and adenosine diphosphate, which in the presence of fibrinogen causes more rapid platelet aggregation. This process may be termed "primary hemostasis" and involves the formation of a temporary hemostatic plug. It is this phase of hemostasis that is measured with a tourniquet test and a bleeding time. It is abnormal in patients who have disturbances of their vasculature or of their circulating platelets and may be accentuated by the ingestion of acetylsalicylic acid (aspirin).

■ **What is Moschcowitz's disease?**

Moschcowitz's disease is also termed "angiopathic thrombohemolytic thrombocytopenia." Of unknown cause, it is associated with damage to tiny vessels resulting in the formation of clots, along with severe hemolytic anemia and profound thrombocytopenia.

■ **What are the stages of coagulation?**

In the intrinsic pathway, the first stage is the formation of plasma thromboplastin. Following either the intrinsic or extrinsic pathway, the second stage is the conversion of prothrombin to thrombin; and the third is the conversion of fibrinogen to fibrin. Stable factor VII is necessary to activate tissue thromboplastin in the extrinsic pathway but is not needed in the intrinsic system.

■ **How is coagulation initiated, following the intrinsic pathway?**

It may be initiated in vivo by the formation of plasma thromboplastin following the release of platelet phospholipids. In vitro, it is initiated by contact with glass. The biochemical approach theorizes that the process is primarily a series of enzyme reactions, each enzyme activating the next ("cascade" or "waterfall" theory). This may be shown diagrammatically according to whether thromboplastin is formed either in vivo or in vitro within the plasma following the intrinsic pathway, or is derived from "tissue juice" outside of the plasma following the extrinsic pathway (see diagram).

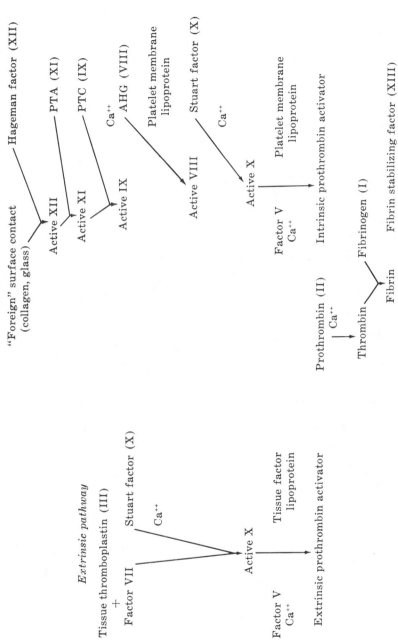

CHAPTER 2

Hematology

THE ERYTHROCYTES
EDWIN L. BEMIS

■ **What is extramedullary hemopoiesis?**

Extramedullary hemopoiesis refers to production of blood cells by organs other than the bone marrow, notably the spleen. It may occur whenever the bone marrow is replaced by abnormal tissue (e.g., in "myelosclerosis with myeloid metaplasia") or whenever the bone marrow fails to supply an increased demand for cells.

■ **What is the function of erythrocytes?**

Erythrocytes provide suitable vehicles for the synthesis, transport, and protection of hemoglobin molecules, which are capable of accepting, transporting, and delivering oxygen to all tissues of the body.

■ **What are the basic elements required for hemoglobin synthesis?**

Protoporphyrin III; an adequate amount of iron in a usable form; "hemopoietic factors" (vitamin B_{12}, folate, vitamin C, hormones) for normal orderly cell maturation; and globin with the necessary polypeptide chains are the elements required for hemoglobin synthesis.

■ **What are some disease states that may be associated with variations in the erythrocyte sedimentation rate?**

In polycythemia with a high volume of packed red cells, the sedimentation rate is extremely slow as it is in the blood of the newborn infant; slow rates are characteristically found in sickle cell anemia as well. Increased rates of sedimentation are found in the presence of increased quantities of proteins of high molecular weight, such as fibrinogen in association with various inflamma-

6

tory processes, or in dysproteinemia (e.g., with plasma cell myeloma).

■ **What are the morphologic principles for the maturation of hemopoietic elements?**

The morphologic principles for the maturation of hemopoietic elements are reduction in the size of the cell as well as its nucleus, loss of nucleoli, and signs of differentiation (hemoglobin formation and extrusion of nucleus in erythrocytes or segmentation of nuclei with formation of specific granules in the cytoplasm of granulocytes).

■ **What are some of the tests that may be altered "fictitiously" by recent blood transfusions?**

Donor red cells may alter any test which is dependent upon examination of the patient's own red cells alone: for example, hemoglobin electrophoresis, the 1-minute alkali denaturation test for fetal hemoglobin, tests for G-6-PD deficiency, pyruvic kinase deficiency, and so on.

■ **How long after a blood transfusion may the bone marrow in pernicious anemia convert from a megaloblastic to a normoblastic character?**

This usually occurs within several hours; this is also the case following an injection of vitamin B_{12}.

■ **What are the cellular structural elements concerned with hemoglobin synthesis?**

The mitochondria are involved in porphyrin synthesis and heme is formed with the incorporation of iron from ferritin aggregates in the cell; globin synthesis takes place in the ribosomes of the endoplasmic reticulum.

■ **What laboratory features may lead poisoning have in common with porphyria?**

The excretion of delta aminolevulinic acid, porphobilinogen, and other abnormal porphyrins, along with protoporphyrin fluorescence of erythrocytes, are some manifestations of lead poisoning.

■ **What are some of the likely diagnoses in a patient having normocytic, normochromic anemia and an elevated platelet count?**

Acute blood loss and an underlying malignancy are probably the most commonly encountered conditions.

■ **What do you know about the iron-binding capacity of blood?**

Normally, iron-binding protein is present in quantities sufficient to bind about 300 μg of iron per 100 ml plasma; usually this is only one-third saturated with iron. Serum iron concentration shows a distinct diurnal variation (highest in the morning and lowest in the late evening) in the normal person, but this variation is minimal in the presence of a hematologic disorder. Iron-binding capacity is remarkably constant in the normal person.

■ **What is the difference between hemosiderosis and hemochromatosis?**

The presence of large amounts of storage iron in body tissues, unattended by tissue damage, is called "hemosiderosis." "Hemochromatosis" is a disorder in which excessive amounts of iron in the body are associated with damage to the tissues, frequently resulting in cirrhosis of the liver and diabetes mellitus.

■ **What amount of hemoglobin may be synthesized from normal body iron stores?**

When iron metabolism is normal, adult body stores are usually sufficient for the synthesis of about 210 gm of hemoglobin or about 1,500 ml of blood.

■ **What is "anemia?"**

Anemia is a condition in which there is a reduced concentration of hemoglobin in the peripheral blood, with an associated decrease of oxygen-carrying capacity and symptoms resulting therefrom. Anemia is not always attended by a reduction in the number of circulating erythrocytes.

■ **What may cause an anemia associated with microcytic, hypochromic red cells and a normoblastic bone marrow?**

The cause may be an iron deficiency state, most commonly associated with chronic blood loss in patients from the United States. Newborns have an increased need for iron, particularly during the first 6 months of life and, unless given supplements, are also prone to develop this form of anemia.

■ **What is "pyridoxine-responsive anemia?"**

Pyridoxine-responsive anemia is a microcytic, hypochromic anemia associated with adequate iron storage and elevated serum iron, which responds to pyridoxine (vitamin B_6) therapy.

■ **What is "hemopoietic principle?"**

It is that substance required for the normal, orderly maturation of blood cells, including those of the myeloid and megakaryocytic series as well as red cells. The major factors embodied in "hemopoietic principle" include vitamin B_{12} and folic acid. A deficiency of either factor may produce megaloblastic dyspoiesis and pancytopenia.

■ **What is pernicious anemia?**

Pernicious anemia is the hereditary lack of "intrinsic factor" in the stomach, which is necessary for absorption of vitamin B_{12} in the ileum; it may be associated with "subacute combined degeneration" of the spinal cord, as well as megaloblastic dyspoiesis of the bone marrow and pancytopenia.

■ **What is the Schilling test?**

It is a test for pernicious anemia. Individuals with this disease will not absorb an appreciable amount of an oral dose of radioactive vitamin B_{12} without the prior addition of intrinsic factor.

■ **How is folic acid formed in the body?**

Most is formed by intestinal bacterial biosynthesis, but conjugase enzymes will also split conjugates of the substance in food (particularly green, leafy vegetables) for absorption.

■ **Why is it important to note the presence of hypersegmented neutrophils?**

This may be the first sign of the development of a megaloblastic process in the marrow, particularly in macrocytic anemia of pregnancy.

■ **Can parasitic infestation result in megaloblastic dyspoiesis?**

Yes, notably the presence of *Dibothriocephalus latus* (fish tapeworm) infestation.

■ **When can "macrocytosis" be seen, unassociated with a true macrocytic anemia?**

Macrocytosis is seen as a "normal" finding in the blood of newborn infants; it is artificially produced by making a blood smear on a nonwettable surface (e.g., siliconized); and appears when many reticulocytes are present, since reticulocytes are larger than older red blood cells.

■ **What are the normal dimers of globins?**

$\alpha_2 \beta_2$ (hemoglobin A_1); $\alpha_2 \gamma_2$ (hemoglobin F); and $\alpha_2 \delta_2$ (hemoglobin A_2).

■ **What is a specific characteristic of fetal hemoglobin?**

It is alkali-resistant (because it contains residues of isoleucine). It is also resistant to oxygen reduction.

■ **What elements are necessary to protect hemoglobin from the effects of oxidant drugs?**

Glucose-6-phosphate dehydrogenase and reduced glutathione

are particularly necessary. Deficiency of either one will result in hemolysis and methemoglobinemia upon exposure to oxidant drugs.

■ **Will a deficiency of pyruvic kinase in red blood cells lead to methemoglobinemia?**

No. It may result in a nonspherocytic, hemolytic anemia unattended by methemoglobinemia.

■ **What is the fate of old red cells that break down within the bloodstream?**

Hemoglobin is released and becomes bound at once to a plasma alpha-2 globulin termed "haptoglobin," which prevents renal excretion; this is then taken up by phagocytic R.E. cells for processing in the usual manner. Haptoglobin is normally present in quantities sufficient to bind about 50 to 150 mg of free hemoglobin per 100 ml plasma.

■ **What is hemolytic disease?**

Hemolytic disease is any disorder in which the red cell life-span is shorter than normal.

■ **What is compensated hemolytic disease?**

The increased rate of destruction is compensated for by augmented erythropoiesis and there is no anemia.

■ **What is hemolytic anemia?**

When augmented red cell production is unable to compensate for the increased rate of destruction, anemia develops. Normal marrow cannot increase its effective output of hemoglobin over 6 to 8 times that of usual, so that when erythrocyte survival is reduced to 15 to 20 days ($\frac{1}{6}$ to $\frac{1}{8}$ of normal), anemia develops and many biochemical changes can be predicted.

■ **What is the most commonly used method for determining red cell life-span?**

The most common method is one in which red cells are drawn from a patient, "tagged" with radioactive chromium, either autotransfused or transfused into a compatible recipient, and the rate of disappearance determined by the fall in degree of radioactivity. Normal "T$\frac{1}{2}$," or time for half of the radioactivity to disappear, is 25 to 35 days, depending upon the anticoagulant used; this is not the expected "half-life" of 60 days, because of elution of chromium and loss of the tracer through the urine at about 1% per day after the first 24 hours. Gastrointestinal blood loss can also be quantitated by this method.

Hemoglobin D and hemoglobin G are also fairly common; they have the same migration on electrophoresis as hemoglobin S at a high pH but may be separated at pH of 6, utilizing citrate agar. Hemoglobin D is probably more common in the American Negro than has been heretofore known. Hemoglobin D is seen in people from India and the British Isles particularly. Hemoglobin E has an incidence as high as 12% in people from Southeast Asia. This results from lysine replacement of glutamic acid in residue No. 26 of the beta chains. Hemoglobin E has the same electrophoretic mobility at pH 8.6 on cellulose acetate as hemoglobin A_2, C, and O.

■ **What is the worldwide distribution of thalassemia?**

Although called "Mediterranean anemia," the disease occurs not only in Southern Europe but in Northern Africa, Asia, and other parts of the world. In the United States it occurs most commonly in Negroes, with or without an associated hemoglobinopathy.

■ **How do paroxysmal nocturnal hemoglobinuria and paroxysmal cold hemoglobinuria differ?**

PNH erythrocytes are particularly susceptible to an acid environment, with hemoglobinuria occurring after awakening from sleep. This is an acquired defect of erythrocytes. PCH is associated with an extracorpuscular abnormality, in which a "Donath-Landsteiner" hemolysin is fixed to RBC's at low temperatures, with hemolysis occurring upon return to a warm environment.

■ **What is cold hemagglutinin disease?**

This is an autoimmune hemolytic disorder associated with high titers of cold agglutinins. It may occur transiently, as in association with *Mycoplasma* pneumonia, or in a more chronic, idiopathic form.

■ **What is autoimmune hemolytic disease of "warm antibody type?"**

Hemolytic disease associated with a positive direct Coombs test is called the "warm antibody type." This is most often associated with another disease entity such as chronic lymphocytic leukemia, malignant lymphoma, or disseminated lupus erythematosus.

■ **What are "Heinz body anemias?"**

Heinz body anemias are hemolytic disorders associated with coccoid, Heinz bodies in the red cells demonstrable with supravital preparations. These can also be visualized by phase-contrast microscopy but are not stained with the usual Romanowski dyes. They represent intracellular precipitations of denatured hemoglobin. They may occur in normal persons (less than 1%) and are more obvious when the spleen is absent. Increased susceptibility to Heinz body formation may be seen in association with defects in the activity of one of the normal red cell enzymes, such as in G-6-PD deficiency; in association with defects in the rate of synthesis or in the structure of the hemoglobin molecule, such as in alpha-thalassemia; or in other conditions related to the presence of unstable hemoglobin molecules.

■ **What is "cardiac hemolytic disease?"**

This is a hemolytic disease associated with a cardiac defect. It is most commonly seen following replacement of heart valves, with hemolysis occurring because of trauma to RBC's in passage through the prosthetic valve. Hemoglobinuria is usually a prominent feature.

■ **What are the anemias of "bone marrow failure?"**

Those associated with "ineffective erythropoiesis," wherein the bone marrow is unable to deliver cells to the peripheral blood. This includes "aplastic" anemia, which is usually associated with leukopenia and thrombocytopenia; "hypoplastic" anemia, which is a term usually applied when there is a pure red cell defect; "sidero-achrestic" anemias, which are associated with large amounts of nonhemoglobin iron in erythrocyte precursors, large iron stores, and high serum iron levels (some such cases are responsive to pyrodoxine therapy); anemias caused by "metabolic inhibition" of the bone marrow, as seen in association with cancer, severe infection, or kidney or liver disease; and so-called "myelophthisis," in which there is abnormal tissue in the bone marrow such as cancerous tissue, the fibrous tissue of "myelofibrosis," inflammatory tissue associated with tuberculosis, and so on. "Myelophthisis" is often associated with marked hemopoiesis in extramedullary sites such as the spleen; only about 50% of such cases show anemia. The most characteristic finding is the presence of nucleated RBC's and a few immature leukocytes in the peripheral blood, which has led to the term "leukoerythroblastosis."

■ **What is polycythemia?**

Polycythemia is a term used to indicate an increased concentration of RBC's in the peripheral blood to above the excessive limits of normal (over 5.7 million/mm^3 for females or 6.4 million/mm^3 for males). "Relative" polycythemia refers to an apparent increase in the peripheral red blood cells caused by a decrease of plasma volume as with dehydration. "True" (absolute) polycythemia refers to an increase of total blody hemoglobin–red cell mass. This may be secondary to an underlying disease or may be primary (idiopathic). When secondary to another disease state, "erythrocytosis" is probably a better term to apply since it is usually associated with only increase of hemoglobin and red cell mass; about 98% of such cases result from decreased oxygen saturation of arterial blood, as with high altitude or disease of lungs or heart. Primary polycythemia (rubra vera) is a "panmyelosis" with abnormal proliferation of megakaryocytes, granulocytic and erythroid cells in the marrow, and increased numbers of all three cell types in the peripheral blood. Arterial oxygen saturation is normal and there is no increased amount of erythropoietin in the blood.

■ **What is DiGuglielmo's disease?**

This refers to a "pure" erythroblastic malignant proliferation. There are bizarre "megaloblastoid" cells in the marrow and many nucleated red blood cells in the peripheral blood (usually over 10 per 100 WBC's). *DiGuglielmo's syndrome* refers to a malignant erythroblastic proliferation combined with maligant proliferation of another cell type (e.g., myeloid: "erythroleukemia").

■ **What is a likely diagnosis in a patient having 1.4 million RBC's, 4.8 gm hemoglobin, 3,800 WBC's, 14,000 platelets, and a reticulocyte count of 0.5%?**

The most likely diagnosis is a macrocytic anemia associated with megaloblastic dyspoiesis of the bone marrow and decreased numbers of all three cellular elements in the peripheral blood. Most often this is associated with pernicious anemia or a folic acid deficiency state.

■ **What are some of the likely diagnoses in a patient having a normocytic, normochromic anemia and an elevated platelet count?**

The most probable include acute blood loss and malignancy.

■ **In what condition may the mean corpuscular hemoglobin concentration go above the normal value?**

In hereditary spherocytosis; unlike mean corpuscular hemoglobin, MCHC is not increased in pernicious anemia.

■ **What is the usual erythrocyte sedimentation rate in sickle cell anemia?**

The rate is very slow, not unlike that seen in polycythemia.

THE LEUKOCYTES

ALFRED MEYERS

■ **List and describe the usual white blood cell types seen in the peripheral blood.**

There are five different leukocyte types: neutrophilic granulocytes, eosinophilic granulocytes, basophilic granulocytes, monocytes, and lymphocytes. The neutrophilic granulocytes usually have a segmented or filamented nucleus. A few less mature forms have a band- (or stab-) shaped nucleus and comprise about 5% or less of the neutrophils. Lymphocytes can be divided into a small and large subtype. The former comprise about 80% of the lymphocytes. (Your description should be compared with the detailed morphology of these cell types which can be found in standard atlases of morphology.)

■ **Where are these cell types formed?**

The granulocytes (the neutrophils, eosinophils, and basophils) are formed in the bone marrow. Monocytes are formed in the reticuloendothelial system including the bone marrow. Lymphocytes originate from lymphoid tissue, which is widely distributed throughout the body. Lymphoid tissue is found in the gastrointestinal tract, respiratory tract, and oropharynx. The oropharynx includes the tonsils and adenoids. Lymph nodes are localized throughout the body and represent drainage points for lymphatics should a foreign antigen spread beyond local tissue sites. The spleen has abundant lymphoid tissue and is a major blood filtering organ. The embryologic origin of the small and large lymphocytes is different, and there are functional differences as well. The thymus is a lymphoid-rich organ responsible for populating lymphoid tissues with small lymphs which are also called T-lymphocytes. In childhood the thymus is a prominent organ in the upper anterior chest but involutes markedly in early adult life. The bone marrow contains lymphoid tissue. In the embryo, it populates lymphoid tissues with large lymphocytes called B-lymphocytes.

■ **Discuss the function of each type and subtype of the leukocytes. Indicate the life-span of each.**

The neutrophilic granulocyte is a phagocytic cell. The neutrophilic granules are microbiocidal proteins. The less conspicuous fine azurophilic granules are rich in enzymes (i.e., lysozyme, peroxidase, hydrolase). After phagocytosis, the granules empty into the phagocytic vacuoles, which form a phagolysosome.

The specific function of the eosinophilic granules is not clear. They apparently contain profibrinolysin. These cells are prominent in inflammations associated with allergy and parasitic infestations. The cells are thought to be chemotactic for fibrin and antigen complexed with IgE. The basophilic granulocyte is rich in histamine and heparin. Histamine has vasodilatory effects. Heparin maintains the fluidity of blood. Both these effects are important in the inflammatory response. IgE is bound to basophils (and its tissue counterpart, the mast cell). Reaction with the specific antigen (allergen) causes degranulation.

The neutrophil, eosinophil, and basophil are short-lived cells, probably surviving several days or less. Activation of the neutrophil hastens its demise.

The monocyte, like the neutrophilic granulocyte, is primarily phagocytic. It sweeps up the debris of the neutrophilic encounter. It is a more effective phagocyte against foreign debris and certain microorganisms. It is important in antigen processing and antigen-antibody complex digestion. The cell has regenerative capacity and is apparently long-lived.

Lymphocytes confer specific immunity. Previous experience with foreign antigens results in enhanced activity, even decades after the primary exposure. Appropriately stimulated, the B-lymphocytes will transform to secretory plasma cells. These secrete specific immunoglobulins. The small or T-lymphocyte is a cell that participates in graft rejection reactions and has certain tumoricidal properties as well as antimicrobial properties. In contrast to the B-lymphocytes, there is no macromolecular immunoglobulin secretion.

The T-lymphs have certain properties or factors probably related to polypeptide formation. These can be demonstrated to transfer immunity, cause migratory inhibition of mononuclear cells, and have cytotoxic properties. The T-lymphocyte readily responds to the stimulation of the mitogen phytohemagglutinin; the B-lymphocyte shows little or no response.

Lymphocyte survival may be quite long-lived. The transformed or reactive lymphocytes may have a reduced survival, particularly the B-lymphocyte. A subpopulation of long-lived or memory B- and T-lymphocytes would account for the anamnestic response.

■ **How may the white blood count and percent differential lead to erroneous interpretation?**

A report of the total leukocyte concentration and its differential by percent must be corrected to absolute concentration for each of the components. Errors in calculations and failure to remember normal absolute concentration may lead to improper identification of specific population shifts. Increases in the concentration for the cell type or types implies (ordinarily) a need for their specific cellular defenses (i.e., neutrophilic phagocytosis). Decreases also must be explained by consideration of such factors that may affect cell production, release, and survival. The following are *approximate* adult normal values that can be used to determine shifts in leukocyte populations:

Neutrophils	2,500-7,500	(with approximately 5% or less bands)
Eosinophils and basophils	50-500	(eos./basos., approximately 5:1)
Lymphocytes	1,000-4,000	(T's/B's, approximately 4:1)
Monocytes	60-600	

Example 1

WBC 20,000/mm³	Percent differential	Absolute concentration/mm³	Change
Neutrophils	70 (12 bands)	14,000	Moderate increase
Eos./Basos.	5	1,000	Slight increase
Lymphocytes	15	3,000	None
Monocytes	10	2,000	Moderate increase

Interpretation: Phagocytic activity increased such as may be seen with bacterial infection and myocardial infarction.

Example 2

WBC 20,000/mm³	Percent differential	Absolute concentration/mm³	Change
Neutrophils	20	4,000	None
Eos./Basos.	2	400	None
Lymphocytes	70	14,000	Marked increase
Monocytes	8	1,600	Mild increase

Interpretation: Lymphocytosis predominates with need for specific immunity such as may be seen with viral infections or certain bacterial infections such as whooping cough.

Example 3

WBC 2,500/mm³	Percent differential	Absolute concentration/mm³	Change
Neutrophils	20	500	Marked decrease
Eos./Basos.	2	50	None
Lymphocytes	70	1,750	None
Monocytes	2	50	Slight decrease

Interpretation: Lymphocytosis is relative and not absolute. Neutropenia predominates. This picture may be seen with bone marrow depression (decreased cell production) or severe hypersplenism (decreased neutrophilic survival and sequestration).

■ **Define inflammation and the role of the white blood count and differential in assessing inflammatory conditions.**

Inflammation is the host's cellular and humoral response to cellular and/or tissue injury. Injury may result from the effects of: (1) ischemia, i.e., myocardial infarction; (2) microorganisms, i.e., bacterial pneumonia, infectious mononucleosis; (3) physical agents, i.e., burn trauma; (4) chemical agents, i.e., lead intoxication; (5) immunologic derangements, i.e., autoimmune thyroiditis, glomerulonephritis; or (6) malignancies.

The inflammation is present at the site of injury. The peripheral leukocytic concentration relates to the site of injury and the production centers (bone marrow and lymphoid tissue). Changes or lack of significant changes may be a clue to the nature of injury as well as its intensity. The white blood count and differential generally lack specificity and give only a broad indication of potential diseases. Generally, changes are more dramatic with acute than with chronic disorders. In addition, the white blood cell count and differential are important means by which one may follow the progress of diseases.

■ **Indicate the neutrophilic changes often noted in acute inflammation.**

These changes may be listed as follows:

1. A substantial increase in neutrophilic concentration
2. A significant percentage increase in band forms (a shift to the left)
3. Prominent azurophilic granulation (toxic granulation)
4. Döhle bodies (cytoplasmic RNA)
5. Cytoplasmic vacuoles
6. Degranulation
7. Increased neutrophilic alkaline phosphatase content
8. Nuclear pyknosis

Not all these qualitative changes may be evident. Such changes are helpful in distinguishing the neutrophilic increases of emotional and physical stress from acute inflammation. An unfavorable prognosis may be expected if the neutrophilic response declines with an increasing proportion of bands and the previously described cellular changes become increasingly more pronounced.

■ **What is the Pelger-Huet anomaly? Indicate its significance.**

This autosomal dominant disorder is characterized by abnormal nuclear structure. The chromatin is overly condensed. The majority of neutrophils show decreased segmentation with peanut or pince-nez shaped nuclei resembling band forms. The heterozygotes have normal leukocytic function. If this anomaly is not recognized, a marked shift to the left may be reported and misinterpreted as severe acute inflammation.

■ **Discuss and analyze the following white blood count.**

A 30-year-old male with a palpable left neck mass.

WBC 12,000/mm³	Percent differential	Absolute concentration/mm³	Change
Neutrophils	30	3,600	None
Eos./Basos.	18/2	2,400	Marked increase
Lymphocytes	40	4,800	Slight increase
Monocytes	10	1,200	Slight increase

Eosinophilia predominates. Eosinophilia is generally accompanied by a slight increase of basophils. Mild eosinophilia may be seen in the healing phases of acute inflammation, such as following surgery. More intense eosinophilia is often noted with dermatitis, parasitic infestation, and many allergic disorders. In this case, because of a neck mass that may represent a lymph node tumor, one must consider a lymphoma, particularly Hodgkin's disease. Hodgkin's disease is frequently associated with pronounced eosinophilia, a reflection of the eosinophilic infiltrates in these nodes.

■ **Discuss the following white blood count in a febrile 16-year-old girl with deranged enzyme liver functions, in terms of practical clinical considerations and supportive morphologic alterations in leukocytes.**

WBC 15,000/mm³	Percent differential	Absolute concentration/mm³	Change
Neutrophils	44 (10% stabs)	6,600	Slight shift to left
Eos./Basos.	3	450	None
Lymphocytes	45	6,750	Moderate increase
Monocytes	8	1,200	Mild increase

The predominant change is lymphocytosis, which is often seen in acute viral infections and occasionally in certain specific non-viral infections. Autoimmune disorders may also show lymphocytosis. A prime consideration in this patient would be infectious mononucleosis with complicating hepatitis. A significant number of lymphocytes will be atypical, exhibiting monocytoid and plasmacytoid features. This impression should be confirmed by heterophile antibody study or EB virus titers. If these prove negative, then one must consider other causes of the infectious mononuclear syndrome, such as infectious and serum hepatitis, cytomegalic inclusion disease, and toxoplasmosis.

■ **Discuss the clinical considerations when the only significant change in the white blood count and differential is absolute monocytosis.**

Mild monocytosis is seen in many clinical disorders, and although not to be ignored, it does not lead to specific considerations. When it is moderate or marked, i.e., three-fold or more of the upper normal value, and unaccompanied by other significant shifts in leukocytic population, one should consider certain clinical disorders such as subacute bacterial endocarditis, disseminated tuberculosis, disseminated malignancy, and preleukemia and aleukemia.

■ **Define and discuss leukemoid reactions.**

A leukemoid reaction represents a peripheral blood picture that simulates leukemia. There may be profound leukocytosis, i.e., 50,000 or greater, with one cell type predominating and accompanied by a small but significant percentage of immature precursors of this cell type. Normal or low counts with immature forms also may simulate subleukemia.

Neutrophilic leukemoid reactions generally show "toxic" changes (as outlined under neutrophilic changes often noted in acute inflammation). The alkaline phosphatase content of the neutrophils will be substantially elevated, in contrast to chronic granulocytic leukemia, in which it is usually depressed. Intense eosinophilic reactions are usually reactive and eosinophilic leukemia is rare. The primary underlying disorder should be identified. Marked intense basophilia is usually suggestive of a basophilic variant of chronic granulocytic leukemia. Lymphocytic leukemoid reactions usually result from infections such as infectious mononucleosis, infectious lymphocytosis, and whooping cough. If unsubstantiated by appropriate serologic and bacteriologic studies, bone marrow and lymph node examination may be necessary. Intense monocytosis or monocytic leukemoid reactions, although temptingly suggestive of monocytic leukemia, often prove to be nonleukemia and indicative of a severe systemic disease.

■ **What is the predominant change in the following white blood count? Discuss possible etiologic mechanisms.**

WBC *3,600/mm³*	*Percent* *differential*	*Absolute con-* *centration/mm³*	*Change*
Neutrophils	40	1,440	Moderate decrease
Eos./Basos.	5	180	None
Lymphocytes	45	1,620	None
Monocytes	10	360	None

There is moderate neutropenia. Initial considerations should be divided between causes of diminished leukopoiesis, abnormal cell release mechanisms, and decreased neutrophil survival or sequestration.

Decreased production may be caused by marrow injury. This may be seen with toxicity of overwhelming infection, drug and chemical toxicity, extensive irradiation damage, and extensive metastatic malignancy to bone marrow. Faulty release mechanisms may explain the low normal or mild neutropenia seen in some Negroes. They have normal marrow cellularity. Megaloblastic anemias usually have concomitant neutropenia and thrombocytopenia. The bone marrows are hypercellular and, although maturation is impaired, segmented neutrophils are readily evident.

The neutrophil will show decreased survival in severe infections, endotoxic shock, drug toxicity, and conditions in which autoimmune mechanisms are stimulated against neutrophils. Hypersplenism may be associated with significant sequestration of neutrophils as well as red blood cells and platelets. Transient neutropenia is sometimes seen in the early stage of acute inflammation because of temporary depletion of circulating granulocytes.

■ **Define agranulocytosis and discuss possible etiologic mechanisms.**

In agranulocytosis there is complete absence of circulating granulocytes. This indicates a profound destruction of circulating peripheral neutrophils, or severe marrow damage with impairment of granulopoiesis. The disorder is usually discovered because of severe infection. Exposure to drugs and unusual chemicals or toxins must be determined. Many drugs have a bone marrow suppressive effect, which is manifested overtly with high dosages. A few patients may demonstrate a selective biochemical sensitivity or idiosyncrasy to a drug with specific effects on dividing cells. In these patients normal doses of such a drug will impair granulopoiesis. Occasionally, drugs may induce an autoimmune reaction with the formation of leukoagglutinins. This may result in sudden, profound destruction of the circulating granulocytes.

■ Discuss and comment on the following white blood count in a 3-year-old child with a history of many infections.

WBC 5,000/mm³	Percent differential	Absolute concentration/mm³	Change
Neutrophils	75	3,750	None
Eos./Basos.	3	150	None
Lymphocytes	12	600	Marked decrease
Monocytes	10	500	None

A child normally has a higher absolute lymphocyte count than an adult. Therefore this count indicates severe lymphopenia. This history suggests impaired immunity and probable diminished lymphopoiesis. Because the T-cells comprise about 80% of circulating lymphocytes, T-cell rather than B-cell depression is likely. This defect may be associated with thymic hypoplasia or aplasia and hypoplastic lymph nodes. Unless this is a combined defect, the globulin level should be normal. Most T-cells are capable of interacting directly with sheep erythrocytes with clusters of red blood cells forming about the T-cells, so-called rosette formation. In this case one could expect very little rosette formation. Skin testing for cell-bound immunity should also be impaired.

■ Define and discuss balanced leukopenia.

This is a decrease of neutrophils and lymphocytes and, to a lesser extent, monocytes without significant alteration of their percentage differential. This combined depression could be expected when there is extensive damage to bone morrow and lymphoid tissue. This may be seen with drug therapy, i.e., cancer chemotherapy, and/or extensive irradiation. The disease process itself, i.e., malignancy, for which these modalities are often used, may involve the hemopoietic and lymphoid centers and further contribute to leukopenia. Another cause of balanced leukopenia is lupus erythematosus, a systemic autoimmune disease with effects on leukocytes, erythrocytes, and platelets.

■ Define and discuss pancytopenia.

Pancytopenia is a decreased concentration of circulating leukocytes, erythrocytes, and platelets. This would indicate depressed myelopoiesis (myelo = marrow) or increased destruction or sequestration of all three elements. A few more common causes of impaired myelopoiesis are megaloblastic anemias, extensive irradiation, drug therapy with bone marrow depression, and extensive marrow infiltration with malignancy. Increased destruction of the circulating formed elements may be seen with severe infection, endotoxic shock, and autoimmune disorders such as lupus erythematosus (LE). Hypersplenism may result in significant sequestration of all formed elements.

■ **Why are eosinopenia, basopenia, and monocytopenia given little recognition?**

The normal concentration of these cells is low, such that the differential may fail to reflect significant decreases. Moreover, when decreases are evident, concomitant changes in neutrophils or lymphocytes are more dramatic. Eosinopenia may be seen in hyperadrenalism (Cushing's disease). Monocytopenia is usually overshadowed by neutropenia.

■ **What is the Thorn test?**

This test determines the change of the absolute eosinophil count before and after ACTH stimulation. If there is a substantial drop in eosinophils to at least one-half the preinjection level, it is presumed that the adrenals are capable of secreting adequate corticoids. Adrenocorticoids cause eosinopenia and lymphopenia.

■ **Describe the LE cell and discuss the probable mechanism of its formation.**

The LE cell is usually a neutrophil that is distended by a large, relatively homogeneous, amphophilic mass slightly smaller than the size of the neutrophil. This mass represents phagocytized, altered nuclear material that has interacted with autoimmune antinuclear antibodies and complement. The most significant nuclear antibody is that formed against native DNA. Neutrophils are chemotactic for complement and phagocytize the complex. In patients with LE, this phenomenon can be demonstrated with incubated peripheral blood, particularly when leukocytes are mildly traumatized by straining or whipping to allow exposure of antigenic nuclear material to the autoantibody. Extracellular altered nuclear masses surrounded by neutrophils, so-called rosettes, are often found in patients with LE but are not specific for this disorder.

■ **What is a tart cell?**

This cell is usually a monocyte that has phagocytized nuclear material from damaged or dead cells. The engulfed mass retains basophilia and a nuclear chromatin pattern. Although common in LE, tart cells may be seen with other disorders.

■ **Describe other tests available to document antinuclear antibodies formed in lupus erythematosus.**

Indirect immunofluorescence has been the most popular screening test. It is quite sensitive and can be titered. This method uses a variety of tissues as sources for nuclear antigen, i.e., liver and thymus. Peripheral leukocytes from O negative blood may be used. Other serologic methods that demonstrate anti-DNA have been developed and include latex agglutination tests, precipitin immunodiffusion, and radioimmune assay. The efficacy of therapy will be manifested by decreasing titers of anti-DNA autoantibody. The disease activity is also correlated with complement levels that decline with increasing activity.

■ **Define a myeloproliferative disorder.**

This is an abnormality of marrow tissue in which there is a seemingly *autonomous unrestrained proliferation* of myelopoietic cells. This usually involves one cell line of differentiation: granulocytic, erythrocytic, or megakaryocytic. Occasionally, two or three cell lines are involved. Mature, intermediate, or primitive cells may predominate. Increased numbers of the overproduced cells, as well as lesser numbers of other immature cell forms, spill into the peripheral blood.

■ **Define and discuss chronic myelogenous leukemia.**

This is a myeloproliferative disorder in which there is marked granulopoiesis. The peripheral blood shows a substantial, often profound increase of mature granulocytes with a small percent of less mature forms. Although neutrophils generally predominate, basophils and eosinophils are also increased and occasionally may predominate. Many of these leukemias show little or no alkaline phosphatase content within the cytoplasm of the neutrophil. Many also have a concomitant chromosomal abnormality with a deletion of the long arm of chromosome 22 (the Philadelphia chromosome). These patients may live for several years until acute leukemic transformation or fatal infection occurs.

■ **Define and discuss acute myelogenous leukemia.**

This is a myeloproliferative disorder characterized by marrow hyperplasia and a peripheral blood dominated by immature precursors of the peripheral granulocytes. Either myeloblasts, promyelocytes, or myelocytes may predominate. Anemia and thrombocytopenia are usual. No consistent chromosomal abnormality is evident. The clinical course of this group is usually very rapid, with the patient expiring because of hemorrhagic complications or infection.

■ **What is an Auer rod?**

This is an azurophilic delicate, elongate crystalloid, sometimes seen within the promyelocytes and monoblasts of leukemia cells. It represents an abnormal primary or azurophilic granule.

■ **Define and discuss erythemic myelosis.**

This is a myeloproliferative disorder in which the marrow shows marked erythroblastic proliferation. The peripheral blood contains many erythroblasts. Proerythroblasts and basophilic erythroblasts predominate in acute erythemic myelosis; polychromatophilic and orthochromic erythroblasts predominate in chronic erythemic myelosis. These patients are anemic and often have atypical erythrocytes with megaloblastic forms. Acute erythemic myelosis has a rapidly fatal course. Polycythemia vera, which may be included in this classification, has the least pernicious prognosis.

■ **Define and discuss megakaryocytic myelosis.**

This is a myeloproliferative disorder characterized by excess proliferation of immature megakaryocytes. The cells are often atypical. There is severe thrombocytopenia, and megakaryocytic fragments are often seen within the peripheral blood. The disease is rapidly fatal. Primary thrombocythemia may be included in this classification and is characterized by hyperplasia of mature but atypical megakaryocytes. There is marked thrombocytosis but these thrombocytes are functionally abnormal.

■ **Define and discuss myelofibrosis.**

Myelofibrosis is a myeloproliferative disorder characterized by patchy marrow fibrosis and interspersed panhyperplastic marrow. There is mild to moderate leukocytosis. The peripheral blood contains a small number of nucleated erythrocytes and immature myeloid elements. Platelets are usually increased in number and show variable size with large forms. The erythrocytes show considerable anisocytosis and poikilocytosis with characteristic teardrop forms. This disorder is often difficult to distinguish from chronic granulocytic leukemia. However, the leukocyte alkaline phosphatase is usually increased and there is no associated Philadelphia chromosome.

■ **List and discuss the mixed myeloproliferative disorders.**

Chronic granulocytic leukemia, polycythemia vera, idiopathic thrombocythemia, myelofibrosis, and erythroleukemia may be considered mixed myeloses. In chronic granulocytic leukemia, polycythemia vera, and idiopathic thrombocythemia, the marrow generally shows hyperplasia of all three elements. Predominance of one of the three cell lines, however, usually characterizes the clinical course of the disorder. Polycythemia vera and idiopathic thrombocythemia may transform into chronic granulocytic leukemia or an acute myelosis. Myelofibrosis shows panhyperplasia accompanied by proliferation of stromal reticulum cells with marrow fibrosis and may terminate with blast transformation. The erythroleukemias show a mixed pattern. The peripheral blood and marrow show increases of immature myeloid and erythroblastic elements. These may eventually transform to a uniform acute myelosis. This mixture of patterns and transitions suggests that the myeloproliferative disorders are closely related entities.

■ **Define and discuss myelomonocytic leukemia.**

Both acute and chronic myelomonocytic leukemias may occur. Some are Philadelphia chromosome–positive and have diminished alkaline phosphatase content of neutrophiles. Chronic myelomonocytic leukemia is a variant of chronic granulocytic leukemia. The peripheral blood contains mature granulocytes, an array of immature myelocytes, and a prominent monocytosis, i.e., 25%. The bone marrow is rich in immature myelocytes. Acute myelomonocytic leukemia has marrow and peripheral blood which are comprised chiefly of immature myeloid elements, and in addition primitive reticulohistiocytic cells. The reticulohistiocytic cells resemble monocytes.

■ **Define and discuss monocytic leukemia.**

Acute monocytic leukemia is a monoblastic leukemia. Its course is rapidly fatal. The monoblasts may contain Auer rods. Peripheral blood characterized by substantial increases of mature monocytes is most often a reactive rather than a leukemic condition.

■ **Define and discuss chronic lymphocytic leukemia.**

This is a seemingly autonomous, unrestrained, progressive mature lymphocytosis. Counts may be extremely high, i.e., 100,000 or more. It is accompanied by lymphocytic hyperplasia in lymphoid tissue. In making the peripheral smear, these lymphocytes are traumatized easily and form smudge cells in and near the feather edge. The leukemic lymphocytes are almost always B-cells. Hypogammaglobulinemia and occasionally monoclonal gammopathy may develop. There is an increased association of autoimmune disorders, i.e., rheumatoid arthritis. Autoimmune hemolytic anemia may occur. Although the clinical course is often protracted, life is usually shortened because of increased susceptibility to infection.

■ **Define and discuss acute lymphocytic leukemia.**

This is a seemingly autonomous, unrestrained, progressive lymphocytosis in which the peripheral blood is dominated by lymphoblasts or prolymphocytes. In children, lymphoblastic leukemia is the most common leukemia. Untreated disease is rapidly fatal because of marrow replacement and complicating anemia, hemorrhage, and infection.

■ **Discuss the differentiation of the acute leukemias and indicate pertinent cytochemical studies.**

The distinction between the acute lymphoblastic leukemias and the nonlymphoblastic leukemias is particularly important because in children the former have had encouraging increases in length of survival and possible cures with specific programs of intensive chemotherapy. Characterization of blast forms sometimes may prove difficult with the Romanowsky stain. The different blast types sometimes show specific cytochemical reactions that aid in their differentiation. A small number of cases will fail to react with any of the special stains. Several special stains should be used. The stains more commonly used include: the PAS, peroxidase, sudan black, and esterase reactions. Lymphoblasts may show PAS-positive granules in their cytoplasm; myeloblasts and monoblasts ordinarily do not. The peroxidase and sudan black reactions, although of different nature, give parallel results. Peroxidase activity and sudan black positivity may be seen in the immature myeloid forms; myeloblasts usually do not react. Immature monocytes may be positive, but their reactivity is more diffuse. Lymphoblasts do not have peroxidase activity. Esterase activity is reported to be most active in the monocytic series.

■ **Define subleukemic and aleukemic leukemia.**

Subleukemic leukemia is that point in the clinical course of leukemia in which only a small number of leukemic leukocytes may be found within the peripheral blood. The marrow, however, will contain substantial increases of leukemic cells adequate for diagnosis. Aleukemic leukemia should contain no peripheral leukemic cells but, as in subleukemia, the marrow will contain substantial numbers of leukemic cells. The peripheral blood may show mild leukocytosis, normal numbers of leukocytes, or leukopenia. Anemia and thrombocytopenia are often present. Monocytosis may be noted. It is the unexplained anemia, thrombocytopenia, leukopenia, or monocytosis which may be a clue to the possibility of leukemia. These definitions are applicable generally to acute leukemias, although in theory the chronic leukemias may go through an aleukemia and subleukemia phase.

■ **Define and discuss preleukemia.**

This is a stage in the evolution of leukemia in which there are no clearly recognizable changes within the peripheral blood and/or bone marrow. Hemopoietic changes, when present, are not characteristic or of significant magnitude or specificity to make the diagnosis of leukemia. In preleukemic acute leukemia, these conditions include anemias that may be megaloblastic, sideroblastic, or aplastic; leukopenias; thrombocytopenia; and unexplained monocytosis. Chromosomal studies may prove important since a substantial proportion of these show abnormal karyotypes not unlike those seen in the acute leukemias. The preleukemia phase of the evolving chronic leukemia is often obvious in retrospect. It shows a slowly progressive insidious change characteristic of the disease. Early suspicion of chronic granulocytic leukemia should have chromosomal analysis for the Philadelphia chromosome. Chronic lymphocytic leukemia will usually show disproportionate increases in B-lymphocytes.

■ **Define and discuss the lymphomas.**

Lymphomas are a group of malignancies which involve the parenchymatous elements of lymphoid tissue. They include the primitive reticular or stem cell and its derivatives, the reticulum cell, histiocyte, lymphoblast, and lymphocyte. These malignancies initially form localized tumors which then invade and metastasize (two common clinical tumors are reticulum, or histiocytic cell sarcoma, and lymphosarcoma). These may rarely be associated with leukemic blood dissemination. This is more frequently seen with the lymphosarcomas. The leukemic lymphosarcoma cell usually shows significant morphologic variation, such as folded and creased nuclei, such that it usually can be distinguished from normal and leukemic lymphocytes. The lymphosarcomas may be associated with dysproteinemia, monoclonal gammopathy, and hemolytic anemias.

Hodgkin's disease is a malignant lymphoma with a varied histologic pattern; often there is marked reactive inflammation and scarring. There are malignant cells interspersed in varying numbers. These may be histiocytes or immunoblasts. A characteristic and virtually diagnostic cell, called the Reed-Sternberg cell, is one of the major morphologic criteria of this disorder. This cell is a malignant bilobed or multinucleated cell. Eosinophilia is noted commonly with Hodgkin's disease. As the disease advances, immunity declines, particularly with reduction of T-cells and cell-bound immunity.

■ **Define and discuss plasma cell myeloma.**

This is a malignant tumor of plasma cells which exhibits varying degrees of maturity and atypia. It usually involves the bone marrow, where there are localized and/or diffuse plamsa cell infiltrates. Radiologic examination of the bone often shows characteristic punched out lesions and/or osteoporosis. There may be hypercalcemia. Painful microfractures are common. Most myelomas are differentiated to the extent that there is secretion of excess immunoglobulin. The immunoglobulin is homogeneous and a monoclonal pattern is evident in protein electrophoresis. IgG and IgA and occasionally IgD and IgE may be synthesized. Excessive light chain formation or inability to couple all the light with the heavy chains may result in light chain secretion into the peripheral blood; sometimes, only the light chain of the immunoglobulin molecule is synthesized. In either case, these light chains are filtered through the kidney into the urine as Bence-Jones protein. Atypical plasma globulins, i.e., cryoglobulin, may be formed. Autoimmune anemia may occur. In the peripheral blood smear rouleaux formation is frequently noted. These patients have anemia. As the disease progresses, they become increasingly susceptible to infection. Occasional cases terminate with plasma cell leukemia.

■ **Define and discuss Franklin's heavy chain disease.**

This may be considered a variant of multiple myeloma in which the cells form and secrete a homogeneous heavy chain fraction of the immunoglobulin molecules. The bone marrow will usually show a significant increase of plasma cells and lymphocytes. Lymphoid tissues show similar infiltrates. There is anemia and susceptibility to infection.

■ **Define and discuss Waldenstrom's macroglobulinemia.**

This is an unrestrained progressive proliferation of IgM secretory cells whose morphology is usually intermediate or transitional between lymphocytes and plasma cells. The IgM is homogeneous and forms a monoclonal spike with protein electrophoresis. The infiltrates are noted in lymphoid tissue, but the bone marrow changes may not be as characteristic as in multiple myeloma. Bence-Jones proteinemia is occasionally present. Rouleaux is prominent. Cryoglobulins may be noted. Minor hemorrhages are frequent, presumably caused by interference of platelet function by the excessive concentration of IgM. These patients are anemic because of blood loss as well as decreased erythropoiesis; a hemolytic component may also be evident. There is increased susceptibility to infection. Leukemia may develop.

■ **Define, discuss, and list causes of myelophthic anemia.**

This is an anemia associated with marrow replacement and is sometimes called leukoerythroblastosis. It is associated with characteristic peripheral blood changes. There are small numbers of nucleated erythrocytes and immature myelocytes; the array of these cells is usually inclined to the more mature forms. Red cells show stippling, anisocytosis, and poikilocytosis with teardrop forms. Platelet concentration is variable but, more important, there is variability of size with giant forms. Extramedullary hemopoiesis or myeloid metaplasia may be present, particularly if the marrow involvement is extensive and the clinical course protracted. This occurs at sites in which the embryo participated in blood formation, i.e., spleen, liver.

Disorders that should be considered when the peripheral blood shows myelophthic anemia include metastatic carcinomas, such as breast carcinoma; malignant lymphoreticular disorders, i.e., lymphosarcoma, multiple myeloma; myelofibrosis; histiocytoses of unknown etiology (Letterer-Siwe, eosinophilic granuloma) ; and certain lipid storage diseases with marrow infiltration by lipid-bearing cells.

■ **For each disorder listed, indicate briefly its significance and the cellular changes: Alder-Reilley's anomaly; Chediak's anomaly; May-Hegglin's anomaly; vacuolated lymphocytes.**

Alder-Reilley's anomaly shows intense azurophilic granulation of granulocytes, occasionally of lymphocytes and monocytes. This may be seen alone or in association with hereditary disorders of mucopolysaccharide metabolism, one expression of which is gargoylism. In the mucopolysaccharidoses, one may also see lymphocytes with large purple inclusions within cytoplasmic vacuoles.

Chediak's anomaly shows large, irregular azurophilic lysosomal granules in neutrophils. Eosinophilic and basophilic granules are also abnormal. Lymphocytes and monocytes may contain azurophilic inclusions. This anomaly is associated with a defect in melanin production and albinism. Leukopenia and thrombocytopenia are present. Infections are common and prove fatal in childhood.

May-Hegglin's anomaly shows coarse Döhle bodies in granulocytes, monocytes, and lymphocytes. Mild leukopenia is present. Giant platelets are present and there may be thrombocytopenia. It is an autosomal dominant disorder whose major problem is associated with thrombocytopenia.

Vacuolated lymphocytes may be seen in several disorders. These include juvenile amaurotic idiocy (Tay-Sachs disease) which is a lipidosis associated with abnormal ganglioside metabolism; Niemann-Pick's disease, another lipidosis caused by sphingomyelin accumulation; and glycogen storage disease.

■ **For each disorder listed, indicate briefly its significance and the cellular change: Niemann-Pick's disease and Gaucher's disease.**

Niemann-Pick's disease is a metabolic disorder of sphingomyelin metabolism caused by an abnormality of sphingomyelinase. Large macrophages with abundant foamy cytoplasm form because of the accumulation of sphingomyelin and sterols. The disease is found in children and is associated with mental and physical retardation. Death usually occurs early because of infection.

Gaucher's disease is a metabolic disorder of lipid metabolism caused by an abnormality of beta glycosidase. There is accumulation of cerebroside within macrophages, forming large cells with a striate appearance. The disease may occur in children or adults. In children there is mental retardation.

In both of these disorders, diagnosis may be made presumptively by the characteristic appearances of these lipid-filled cells. The bone marrow is a convenient source of demonstrating these cells.

■ **Discuss the possible cause of chronic granulomatous disease and the nitrobluetetrazolium test.**

This disease is an example of abnormal neutrophilic function without morphologic expression. These patients have recurrent infection, possibly caused by a group of closely related enzymatic disorders, some of which may be sex-linked and occur in males. Phagocytosis is not impaired but there is selective loss of bactericidal activity. The enzymatic defect in the neutrophil is apparently caused by diminished peroxide effectiveness or formation, which is reduced to sublethal levels by catalase-producing organisms. *Staphylococcus aureus, Serratia,* and *Candida* infections are common. This selectivity is apparently a result of catalase activity in these organisms which is protective. In non-catalase producers such as the streptococci, there is adequate bactericidal activity.

This defect can be demonstrated by inducing a burst of oxidative activity. Stimulated granulocytes will reduce NADH. The reduced NADH will interact with the NBT dye, forming a blue formazan compound. NADH reduction is impaired in this disorder and therefore production of the blue formazan dye is reduced. This reaction can be quantitated by supernatant studies or by scoring the granulocytes.

CHAPTER 3

Immunohematology

GORDON LANG

■ **List twenty historical landmarks that have been important to the field of immunohematology.**

1616   William Harvey discovered the circulation of blood.

1656   Sir Christopher Wren injected various medications into the veins of dogs.

1665   Richard Lower performed the first successful transfusion from the carotid artery of one dog into the jugular vein of another dog.

1667   Jean Baptiste Denis performed the first recorded transfusion of a human. Lamb blood was given to a young man.

1818   James Blundell performed the first transfusion of human blood to another human.

1901   Karl Landsteiner discovered ABO blood groups.

1914   L. Agote administered the first transfusion of human blood that utilized sodium citrate as an anticoagulant.

1916   Rous and Turner demonstrated that the addition of dextrose to citrated blood exerted a favorable effect on the preservation of blood.

1937   Fantus opened the first blood bank in the United States. It was located in Chicago at Cook County Hospital.

1940   Landsteiner and Weiner reported the Rh blood factor.

1943   Loutit and Mollison described the use of ACD (acid-citrate-dextrose) solution for the preservation of blood.

1945   Coombs, Mourant, and Race described the use of the anti-human globulin test, which was based upon the observations of Moreschi (1908), for the detection of "incomplete" Rh agglutinins.

1950   Audrey Smith demonstrated that erythrocytes mixed with glycerol could be frozen and thawed without injury.

1952   Jean Dausset described the occurrence of leukocyte iso-antibodies in the serum of patients transfused with blood from many donors. This led to the development and understanding of the HL-A system in relation to survival of organ transplants.

1953 and 1954   Valtis and Kennedy reported a marked shift to the left (decrease P50) occurred in the oxygen-hemoglobin dissociation curve when blood was stored for a week or more in the ACD solution.

1957   Gibson and associates described the use of CPD (citrate-phosphate-dextrose) solution for the preservation of blood.

1958   Dudley and associates described the use of plastic bags for storing and transfusing blood.

1961   Stern first described that passive administration of anti-Rh_o (D) would prevent primary Rh immunization.

1965   Blumberg and associates described the occurrence of the Australia antigen (hepatitis-associated antigen) in patients with hepatitis.

1967   Benesch and Benesch and Chanutin and Curnish independently reported that the shift to the left in the O_2 dissociation curve (decrease P50) which occurs in ACD stored blood resulted from a decreasing concentration of 2,3-diphosphoglycerate (2,3-DPG).

■ **What is an antigen?**

An antigen is any substance (usually protein in nature) which, when introduced into an individual who himself lacks the substance, stimulates the production of an antibody and which, when mixed with the specific antibody, reacts with it in some observable way, such as agglutination, hemolysis, or precipitation.

■ **What is an antibody?**

An antibody is a specific substance (usually a globulin) produced by an individual in response to the introduction of an antigen. The antibody will react specifically with that antigen in some observable way, as described above.

■ **What are hemagglutinogens, hemagglutinins, and isohemag-glutinins?**

Antigens present on the surface of erythrocytes are referred to as hemagglutinogens and antibodies that agglutinate erythrocytes are referred to as hemagglutinins. Isohemagglutinins are antibodies which agglutinate erythrocytes of another member of the same species.

■ **What is isoimmunization?**

Isoimmunization is the formation of immune antibodies by a member of a given species against some antigen normally absent from its own body but present in another member of the same species. Rh_0 (D) positive blood transfused to a Rh_0 (D) negative individual can result in isoimmunization to the Rh_0 (D) isoagglutinogen.

■ **What is a hemolysin?**

A hemolysin is a type of antibody which, in the presence of complement, results in liberation of hemoglobin from the erythrocytes.

■ **What is complement?**

Complement consists of a series of nine plasma components which react sequentially and are necessary to produce hemolysis. According to the World Health Organization nomenclature and reaction sequence, they are C1, C4, C2, C3, C5, C6, C7, C8, and C9. C1 is composed of three subcomponents; C1q, C1r, and C1s. Intermediate complexes formed by the reaction of the erythrocyte and the antibody with the various components are named according to the complement component bond. Calcium and magnesium are required for completion of the reaction sequence and therefore anticoagulants that bind these cations inhibit complement dependent reactions. Heating serum to 56° C for 30 minutes completely inactivates C1 and C2 and partially inactivates C4.

■ **What is agglutination?**

Agglutination is the visible clumping reaction that occurs when suspensions of erythrocytes, latex particles, or bacteria containing specific antigens are mixed with a serum containing specific antibodies for those antigens.

■ **What is the ABO blood group system? Indicate the major groups within this system.**

The ABO blood group system was the first human blood group system discovered. Landsteiner in 1901 found that human blood could be classified into three groups—A, B, and O. One year later

Landsteiner's students, Decastello and Sturli, discovered the group AB. The ABO classification is based upon the presence on the surface of the erythrocyte of either, neither, or both of two antigenic and type-specific polysaccharide substances, A and B. The groups are named for the antigen (agglutinogen) present on the erythrocyte.

Antigen present	Blood group
A	A
B	B
A and B	AB
Neither	O

■ **What is a major difference between the ABO blood group system and the other blood group systems?**

The ABO blood group system is the only system that regularly contains within serum "naturally" occurring antibodies (agglutinins). These agglutinins do not react with the erythrocytes that are suspended in the serum. All of the other blood group systems do not regularly have "naturally" occurring antibodies in the serum. In other systems, antibodies develop secondary to artificial immunization following blood transfusion or pregnancy. The "naturally" occurring antibodies (agglutinins) of the ABO blood group system are:

Blood group	Antibody present
A	Anti-B
B	Anti-A
AB	Neither
O	Anti-A and anti-B

■ **Discuss the cross reacting anti-A, B (C) present in group O serum.**

It is well known that absorption of group O serum with either A or B erythrocytes will reduce the titer of both anti-A and anti-B. This finding led to the discovery that group O serum contains, in addition to anti-A, anti-A_1, and anti-B—anti-A, B (C). Group O serum reacts with all of the various subgroups of A and all B erythrocytes but does not react with O cells. Group O serum must be used to prove that erythrocytes reacting negatively to anti-A and anti-B serum are truly O cells. Certain rare cells that are not O cells (e.g., Ax) will react negatively with anti-A and anti-B serum as do O cells. However, when these cells are reacted with group O serum, agglutination occurs. This reaction is caused by the presence of anti-A, B (C) in the group O serum. It is believed by most investigators that anti-A, B reacts with a portion of the A or B antigen that is in common and therefore cross reacts. Others have proposed the presence of another antigen (C).

■ **What is absorbed B or anti-A$_1$ serum?**

A$_1$ erythrocytes can be easily separated from A$_2$ erythrocytes by reacting them with group B serum which has been absorbed with A$_2$ erythrocytes. This absorption removes anti-A, which reacts with both A$_1$ and A$_2$ cells, but does not remove anti-A$_1$, which reacts only with A$_1$ erythrocytes. Therefore, absorbed B serum will react only with A$_1$ erythrocytes.

■ **What are the subgroups of A?**

In 1911 it was discovered by von Dungern and Hirszfeld that there were subgroups of A or variants of antigen A. Anti-A serum obtained from group B individuals contains two isoagglutinins: anti-A, which reacts with all group A and AB erythrocytes, and another isoagglutinin, anti-A$_1$, which reacts with only about 80% of individuals with group A or AB erythrocytes. Individuals who react with anti-A$_1$ are called A$_1$ and those who do not are called A$_2$.

The practical importance of the A subgroups, A$_1$, A$_2$, A$_1$B, and A$_2$B, is that A$_2$ and especially A$_2$B erythrocytes may react more weakly with anti-A serum than do A$_1$ and A$_1$B erythrocytes, and their detection may be missed. It is also important that about 1% of A$_2$ individuals and 25% of A$_2$B individuals have anti-A$_1$ in their plasma. These individuals cannot be transfused with blood that contains the A$_1$ antigen.

Several other subgroups have been described, namely A$_3$, A$_4$, and A$_x$. These cells generally react weakly or not at all with group B serum. They are all agglutinated by serum from group O individuals. A$_3$ erythrocytes when reacted with group B serum agglutinate in a mixed field pattern, i.e., some cells agglutinate and others do not. A$_m$ cells may react negatively with group O and group B serum. A substances are present in the secretions (saliva, etc.) of these individuals if they are secretors. The reactions of the subgroups are summarized at the top of p. 39.

	Direct grouping						Reverse grouping (cells)			
Phenotype	Anti-A group B serum	Anti-B group A serum	Anti-A₁ absorbed B serum	Lectin Dolichos biflorus	Anti-A, B (C)	Anti-H	A_1	A_2	B	O
A_1	+	−	+	+	+	±	−	−	+	−
A_2	+	−	−	−	+	+	−	−	+	−
A_3	+mf*	−	−	−	+mf*	+mf*	−	−	+	−
A_x (A_4)	−or±	−	−	−	+	+	− or +	−	+	−
A_m	− to vwk*	−	−	−	− to vwk*	+	−	−	+	−

*mf = mixed field; vwk = very weak.

■ **What are agglutinins obtained from plants called?**

Lectins are extracts obtained from certain plants which agglutinate red cells of a particular antigen. Examples are:

Plant	Agglutinin present
Dolichos biflorus	anti-A
Ulex europaeus	anti-H
Iberis amara	anti-M
Vicia graminea	anti-N
Bandeiraea simplicifolia	anti-B
Arachis hypogoea (peanut)	anti-T

Extracts from some snails have anti-A activity

■ **What is H substance? What happens when the gene responsible for H substance is absent?**

Most human erythrocytes contain a basic substance called H substance. This substance, under the influence of the A or B gene, is converted to A or B substance. O erythrocytes contain the largest quantity of H substance and AB the least. The reaction strength of anti-H with various blood groups in descending order is $O > A_2 > A_2B > B > A_1 > A_1B$. Anti-H may be found in the plasma of a rare A_1, A_1B, or B individual whose erythrocytes contain very little H substance.

A very rare individual contains no H or A or B substance on his erythrocytes. The plasma of the individual contains anti-H and anti-A and anti-B. The blood group of this individual is called Bombay or Oh. These individuals lack an H gene which normally converts a basic precursor substance to H substance which in turn is acted upon by A and/or B genes to form A and B substance.

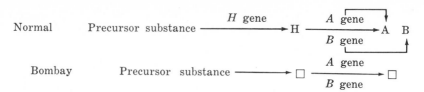

The reactions of group O and group Oh individuals with known antisera and cells are summarized below.

	Direct grouping						*Reverse grouping (cells)*			
Pheno-type	*Anti-A group B serum*	*Anti-B group A serum*	*Anti-A₁ absorbed B serum*	*Lectin Dolichos biflorus*	*Anti-A, B (C)*	*Anti-H*	A_1	A_2	B	O
O	−	−	−	−	−	+	+	+	+	−
Oh	−	−	−	−	−	−	+	+	+	+

Bombay individuals will transmit to their children A and/or B genes if they possess them. A mating between an Oh and an O individual could result in an A or B child.

■ **Compare the immunoglobulins.**

Immunoglobulins are specific proteins produced by the B lymphocytes in response to antigenic stimulation. Five distinct classes of immunoglobulins have been described; IgA, IgG, IgM, IgD, and IgE. The blood group antibodies are associated with the IgA, IgG, and IgM classes.

The basic immunoglobulin molecule consists of two heavy polypeptide chains and two light polypeptide chains. The heavy chains are connected to each other by a disulfide bond, (—S—S—); a light chain is connected to each heavy chain by a similar bond, (—S—S—).

The heavy chains are specific for each class of immunoglobulin, whereas the light chains of the five classes have similar characteristics and have been designated as kappa and lambda. The IgG immunoglobulins have been divided into four subclasses, the IgA into two subclasses.

The immunoglobulins that are produced following initial exposure to a foreign antigen are usually of IgM specificity, whereas during subsequent exposure IgG immunoglobulins are produced. Table 1 summarizes the immunoglobulins.

■ **Discuss the development of the isoagglutinins of the ABO system.**

At birth about 40% of infants have no detectable isoagglutinins

Table 1. Immunoglobulin characteristics

	IgG	IgA	IgM	IgD	IgE
Molecular weight	150,000	150,000	1,000,000	150,000	190,000
Sedimentation constant	7S	7S-18S	19S	7S	8S
Concentration mg/dl (average)					
Adult	1,200	300	100	2	0.03
Cord blood	600	0	10	–	–
Placental transfer	Yes	No	No	No	No
Length	250A		1,000A		
Gm allotype	Yes	No	No	No	No
Inv allotype	Yes	Yes	Yes	Yes	Yes
Erythrocyte agglutination activity	Incomplete	Incomplete	Complete	None	None
Heavy chains	Gamma (γ)	Alpha (α)	Mu (μ)	Delta (δ)	Epsilon (ϵ)
Light chains	Kappa (κ), lambda (λ)	κ, λ	κ, λ	κ, λ	κ, λ
Molecular formula	$\gamma_2\kappa_2$, $\gamma_2\lambda_2$	$(\alpha_2\kappa_2)$ 1-3 $(\alpha_2\lambda_2)$ 1-3	$(\mu_2\kappa_2)$ 5 $(\mu_2\lambda_2)$ 5	$\delta_2\kappa_2$ $\delta_2\lambda_2$	$\epsilon_2\kappa_2$ $\epsilon_2\lambda_2$
Subclasses	$\gamma_{1,2,3,4}$	$\alpha_{1,2}$	$\mu_{1,2}$	—	—
Complement fixation	$\gamma_{1,2,3}$ yes; γ_4 no	No	Yes	?	No

in their serum. The isoagglutinins found in the remaining 60% of infants are passively transferred from the mother and isoagglutinin produced by the infant. The passively transferred isoagglutinin has IgG specificity, whereas the isoagglutinin produced by the infant prior to birth has IgM specificity. Significant levels of the ABO isoagglutinins are detected between 3 and 6 months of age; the maximum titer is attained at 5 to 10 years of age. The ABO isoagglutinins have traditionally been divided into two types, the "naturally occurring" and the "immune occurring" isoagglutinins. The "naturally occurring" isoagglutinins are thought to be produced as an immune response to ingested or inhaled antigenic substances found in nature which are similar to human A and B substances. The "immune occurring" isoagglutinins are found in persons who have been stimulated with A and B substances following incompatible transfusions, heterospecific pregnancies (e.g., O mother, A child), and following injections of soluble blood group substances or other materials such as vaccines which may contain A and/or B sub-

Table 2. Comparison of naturally occurring and immune anti-A

	Natural	Immune
Reacts with saline suspended cells	Yes	No
Anti-human globulin test required to detect	No	Yes
Neutralized by soluble blood group substances (Witebsky substances)	Yes	No
Lyses erythrocytes	Few	Most
Bind complement	Yes	Only IgG, not IgA
Type of immunoglobulin	IgM	IgG or IgA
Heat	Labile	Stable
Reaction with pig A^p cells	No	Yes
Optimal temperature for reaction	Room temp.	37° C

stances. The characteristics of the anti-A naturally occurring and the anti-A immune isoagglutinins are outlined in Table 2.

■ **Discuss the inheritance of the ABO blood group system.**

The ABO blood group of an individual is determined by the genes that he inherits from his parents.

Three allelic genes are responsible for the determination of the ABO genotype. The genes, ignoring the subgroups, are genes *A, B,* and *O.* The *A* and *B* genes give rise to the antigens A and B by converting H substance to A or B agglutinogen. The *O* gene is an amorph (a gene that does not produce any recognizable effect). It does not have any effect upon H substance.

Each individual inherits one *A, B,* or *O* gene from each of his parents. The *O* gene being an amorph and a recessive gene is only detectable in individuals who inherit this gene from both parents. Individuals who inherit only one *O* gene are phenotypically similar to individuals who are homozygous for either the *A* or the *B* gene (e.g., AA, AO; BB, BO).

With rare exceptions the following rules have been postulated for the inheritance of the ABO and other blood group agglutinogens.

1. An agglutinogen cannot be present in the blood of an individual unless it is present in the blood of one or both parents.
2. An individual who is homozygous for an agglutinogen must transmit the gene responsible to all of his children.
3. A child who is homozygous for an agglutinogen must have inherited a gene responsible from both of his parents.

Applying these statements to the ABO group it can be stated that:

1. Agglutinogens A or B cannot be present in the blood of a child unless present in the blood of one or both parents.
2. A group AB parent cannot have a child of group O.
3. A group O parent cannot have a group AB child.

■ **Indicate the ABO phenotypes of children that are possible if the ABO phenotypes of the parents are known.**

Phenotype of parents	Possible phenotypes of children
O + O	O
O + A	A or O
O + B	B or O
A + A	A or O
A + B	A or B or O or AB
B + B	B or O
O + AB	A or B
A + AB	A or B or AB
B + AB	A or B or AB
AB + AB	A or B or AB

■ **What is meant by secretor or nonsecretor status of an individual?**

About 80% of Caucasian individuals contain, within their saliva and other body fluids, H substance. These individuals, if they are also group A, B, or AB, will also have A or B substance in their saliva. The remaining 20% of Caucasian individuals are known as nonsecretors—these substances are not present in their saliva or other body fluids. The secretor status is inherited as a mendelian dominant. The gene responsible for secretor status is called *Se* (allele *se*). Secretors may be of genotype *SeSe* or *Sese,* whereas nonsecretors are of the genotype *sese.*

The A, B, and H substances in body fluids are water soluble. The A, B, and H substances in erythrocytes and other tissues are alcohol soluble, and their presence is not determined by the secretor gene.

The *Se* gene interacts with the Lewis gene *(Le)* so that most secretors of ABH substances are Lewis (Le^a) negative and most nonsecretors of ABH substances are Lewis (Le^a) positive.

■ **How does the Lewis blood group system differ from the other blood group systems?**

The antigens of all blood group systems except the Lewis antigen are an integral part of the red cell membranes. The Lewis antigens are water soluble plasma and salivary antigens that are absorbed onto the surface of the membranes of erythrocytes. Cord blood is generally nonreactive or only very weakly reactive to anti-Le^a or anti-Le^b. Lewis reactivity is not apparent until the infant is several weeks old, at which time the concentration of plasma Lewis substance is adequate for red cell absorption. The Lewis genes are designated as *Le* and *le*. The production of Le^a substance is controlled by the *Le* gene, which is dominant. The *le* gene is an amorph. Le^b substance results from the conversion of Le^a substances under the influence of the *H* and *Se* gene. The A, B, H, and Lewis substances are derived from the same precursor. The interrelationship of the ABO, Lewis, and secretor status can be best briefly explained by Table 3.

The table reveals that individuals in the phenotype Le(a+b−) are nonsecretors of A, B, or H substances. Individuals who are *Se* positive, *Le* positive generally produce insufficient Le^a substance to result in erythrocytes that are Le^a positive and are thus of the phenotype Le(a−b+). Rare O or A individuals may not convert all of the Le^a substance to Le^b substance and thus may have the rare phenotype of Le(a+b+). On the other hand, *Se* positive, *Le* positive individuals of blood group A or B may have erythrocytes that react weakly with anti-Le^b because most of the Le^b substance has been converted to A or B substance.

Le^a substance is not converted to Le^b substance unless an individual possesses both the *H* and the *Se* gene, therefore *H* negative (Bombay, Oh) individuals are either Le(a+b−) or Le(a−b−).

■ **Briefly describe the antibodies of the Lewis system.**

Lewis antibodies are produced by Le(a−b−) individuals without known antigenic stimulation. Lewis substances are thought to be ubiquitous. The antibodies of this system are IgM and all have the ability to bind complement. Reactivity of most Lewis antibodies is best below room temperature, with some reacting at 37° C and with non gamma anti-human globulin serum.

Several varieties of Lewis antibodies have been described. Anti-Le^a, the most common, is found in about 12% of Le(a—b—) individuals. All individuals with this antibody have at least one *Se* gene and therefore secrete ABH substance. There is a decreased incidence of the group O genotype in individuals with anti-Le^a. Anti-Le^b is at times found as a weak antibody in serums that con-

Table 3. Schematic of the ABO, Lewis, and secretor interrelationships

	Substances in saliva	Lewis pheno-type RBC's	Incidence	
			Caucasian	Negro
Precursor substances →(le gene)→ [PS] →(Se gene / H gene)→ [H] →(A gene / B gene)→ [A B]	ABH	Le(a−b−)	3%	17%
→(Le gene / H gene / Se gene)→ [Leª] → [Leᵇ] + [H] →(A gene / B gene)→ [A B]	A, B, H, Leª, Leᵇ	Le(a−b+)	74%	55%
[Leª] →(H gene / se gene)→ [Leª] →(A gene Ineffective / B gene)	Leª	Le(a+b−)	23%	22%
le gene → [PS] →(H gene / se gene)→ [PS] →(A gene Ineffective / B gene)	—	Le(a−b−)	0.6%	6%

A, B, H, Leª, and Leᵇ substances in body fluids are water soluble and their presence is determined by the secretor gene.
A, B, and H substances in erythrocytes and other tissue are alcohol soluble and their presence is not determined by the secretor gene.

tain potent anti-Le^a. Individuals who produce pure anti-Le^b are of the phenotype Le(a—b—) and do not possess any *Se* genes, and therefore do not secrete ABH substances. Two types of anti-Le^b have been described; one, designated as anti-Le^{bL}, reacts with Le^b positive cells of groups A, B, O, and AB; the other, designated as anti-Le^{bH}, reacts only with Le^b positive cells of group O individuals. Several other antibodies have been described that react only with Le(a—b—) cells of various secretor status.

■ **Describe the two major theories of inheritance of the Rh blood group system.**

The Fisher-Race theory of inheritance suggests that there are three pairs of allomorphic genes: *C, c; D, d;* and *E, e*. Three of these genes are present, closely linked at separate loci, on each of a pair of chromosomes. It was proposed that each gene is responsible for producing antigenic material capable of stimulating agglutinins. To date, no antibodies to —d— have been identified.

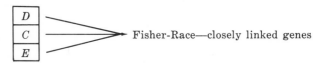

The Weiner theory postulates that there are eight standard allelic genes, one gene located at a single locus on each of a pair of chromosomes. The Weiner genes are R^0, R^1, R^2, R^z, r, r', r'', r^y. Each of these genes is responsible for the production of complex antigens which have several different serologic specificities called factors. The corresponding Weiner genes, antigens, and factors and Fischer-Race genes and antigens are compared in Table 4.

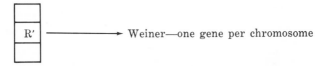

■ **Discuss the nomenclature of the Rh blood group system; include phenotypes, genotypes, and gene frequency.**

Two distinctly different nomenclatures have evolved; one is based on the Weiner theory of inheritance of the Rh antigenic determinants, and the other on Fisher-Race theory. Both nomenclatures are widely used and the blood bank technologist must be familiar with both. Table 4 gives the corresponding equivalent terms for both nomenclatures. The numbers to the right of the

Table 4. Comparison of Weiner and Fisher-Race nomenclatures

Genes			Weiner antigens (8)	Weiner factors (6)		Fisher-Race antigens (6)	
Weiner (8)		Fisher-Race (6)					
R^0 .027	c D e	.027	Rh_0	hr' Rh_0 hr"	.80 .85 .97	c D e	.80 .85 .97
R^1 .41	C D e	.41	Rh_1	rh' Rh_0 hr"	.70 .85 .97	C D e	.70 .85 .97
R^2 .15	c D E	.15	Rh_2	hr' Rh_0 rh"	.80 .85 .30	c D E	.80 .85 .30
R^z .002	C D E	.002	Rh_z	rh' Rh_0 rh"	.70 .85 .30	C D E	.70 .85 .30
r .38	c d e	.38	rh	hr' Hr_0 hr"	.80 .63 .97	c d e	.80 .63 .97
r' .006	C d e	.006	rh'	rh' Hr_0 hr"	.70 .63 .97	C d e	.70 .63 .97
r" .005	c d E	.005	rh"	hr' Hr_0 rh"	.80 .63 .30	c d E	.80 .63 .30
r^y .0001	C d E	.0001	rh^y	rh' Hr_0 rh"	.70 .63 .30	C d E	.70 .63 .30

genes, antigens, and factors are the frequencies of these in Caucasians. These are used to calculate genotype frequency.

Phenotype is defined as the observable reaction or characteristics of an individual. The Rh phenotype is determined by observing the reactions of the five standard antisera: anti-Rh_0 (D), anti-rh' (C), anti-rh" (E), anti-hr' (c), and anti-hr" (e). The Fisher-Race phenotype is written by observing cell reaction with these sera and first writing the C's, then D's, and finally the E's to indicate the antigens present, e.g., CcDEe. The Weiner phenotype is more difficult as it requires memorization of the Weiner antigens as determined by the reactions with the three Rh antisera and the two hr antisera, e.g., Rh_0rh (Fisher-Race phenotype ccDee). If the Rh_0 (D) factor is present, list the corresponding Weiner antigen first, e.g., Rh_0rh. Rh is only used when the Weiner Rh_0 (D) factor is included in the Weiner antigen. If the Rh_0 (D) factor is absent, the symbol rh is utilized. Subscripts 1, 2, and Z and superscripts ', ", and y are used to indicate the presence of the other blood factors, rh', rh", and rh'rh", e.g., Rh_2rh^y. Genotype refers to the genes possessed by an individual for a particular trait. The Fisher-Race Rh genotype can be estimated from the phenotype with some degree of accuracy by examining the phenotype and making sets of genes listing all possible combinations. Assign one set to the left and one set to the right of a slash mark, e.g., CDe/cde. If D is present in one set and not in the other, the set with the D should be to the left of the slash. The possible genotypes in an individual with phenotype CCDEe are CDE/CDe, CDE/Cde, and CDe/CdE.

The Weiner Rh-Hr genotype is determined by listing all of the Weiner gene combinations possible from inspection of the phenotype. In heterozygote Rh_0 individuals the gene containing the Rh_0 factor should be given first, e.g., R^1r. The capital R indicates that the gene has the Rh_0 blood factor and the lower case r indicates that the Rh_0 blood factor is not present. Superscripts 1, 2, Z, ', ", and y are used to designate the presence of other blood factors rh', rh", rh'rh". No subscripts and no h's are used in genotype designation. The possible genotypes in an individual of phenotype Rh_zRh_1 (CCDEe) are R^ZR^1, R^Zr', and R^1r^y.

The determination of the most probable genotype is important in the proper antenatal evaluation of possible hemolytic disease of the newborn. All children of a homozygous Rh_0 (D) father will have the Rh_0 factor, whereas only 50% of the children of a heterozygous Rh_0 (D) father and Rh_0 (D) negative mother will have the factor.

The most probable genotype is determined by determining the frequencies of the various genotypes. The genotype with the highest frequency is the most probable genotype. The calculation of genotype frequencies is simple. The frequency of a genotype with two like genes, e.g., rr, is the square of the gene frequency.

Frequency of r gene is 0.38
∴ Frequency of genotype rr is:
0.38² or 0.38 × 0.38 = 0.144
0.144 × 100 = 14.4%

The frequency of a genotype with two unlike genes is twice the product of the gene frequencies.

Frequency of r gene is 0.38
Frequency of R^1 gene is 0.41
$\therefore$ Frequency of genotype $R'r$ is:
  $2 \times 0.38 \times 0.41 = 0.312$
  $0.312 \times 100 = 31.2\%$

■ **What is the numerical system of designating the Rh-Hr blood group?**

A third method of identifying the Rh-Hr blood factors has been described by Rosenfield. Each Rh factor is designated by number. The phenotype Rh_2rh(ccDEe) would be written Rh: 1, -2, 3, 4, 5. The numbers corresponding to Weiner factors and Fisher-Race antigens are given in Table 5.

■ **What is the D^u ($\Re h_0$) variant?**

D^u ($\Re h_0$) is an Rh antigen that reacts weakly or not at all with the usual saline and/or slide anti-Rh_0 (D) sera. Those that react weakly are referred to as "high grade" D^u and those that are non-reactive and require anti-human globulin sera for their detection are called "low grade" D^u.

Some of the so-called high grade D^u's result from a gene interaction effect exerted by the presence of the r' *(Cde)* gene upon the gene on the opposite chromosome which determines Rh_0 (D). This gene interaction results in a suppressed reactivity of the Rh_0 (D) antigen.

The remaining "high grade" and "low grade" D^u's ($\Re h_0$) are genetically weak antigens that are passed from one generation to another. According to the Weiner theory the Rh_0 (D) factor is composed of four components, Rh^A, Rh^B, Rh^C, and Rh^D. The lack of one or more of these components results in a weak reacting $\Re h_0$ variant, the so-called D^u ($\Re h_0$).

■ **What is the G antigen of the Rh system and what is its significance?**

Table 5. Comparison of Weiner, Fisher-Race, and Rosenfield nomenclatures

Weiner factors	Fisher-Race antigen	Rosenfield numbers
Rh_0	D	Rh_1
rh'	C	Rh_2
rh"	E	Rh_3
hr'	c	Rh_4
hr"	e	Rh_5

The G, rh^G, or Rh_{12} antigen is virtually present on all erythrocytes that are C (rh') positive and/or D (Rh_0) positive.

Most sera that are thought to contain anti-C (rh') and anti-D (Rh_0) actually are comprised of anti-D (Rh_0) and anti-G (rh^G) or anti-D (Rh_0), anti-C (rh'), and anti-G (rh^G). These facts have explained the apparent formation of anti-CD in cde/cde (rr) mothers whose husbands and babies are D (Rh_0) positive, C (rh') negative. In reality the antibody is anti-D (Rh_0) and anti-G (rh^G) rather than anti-D (Rh_0) and anti-C (rh').

■ **Discuss the LW antigen.**

LW is a high-incidence antigen found on the erythrocytes of humans and monkeys and not present on the cells of rabbits and guinea pigs. LW stands for Landsteiner and Weiner; they were the first to produce antibodies to this antigen in animals. Antibodies to this antigen are produced in rabbits and guinea pigs when immunized with human or monkey erythrocytes. A few LW negative individuals with anti-LW have been found. The gene (LW) responsible for LW antigen is independent of the genes responsible for Rh antigens. The production of LW and Rh antigens, however, requires common precursor substances. All individuals without detectable Rh antigens, Rh null, have to date been LW negative. LW negative individuals may have a normal Rh antigen composition or may be Rh null. Giblett has proposed the following genetic pathway.

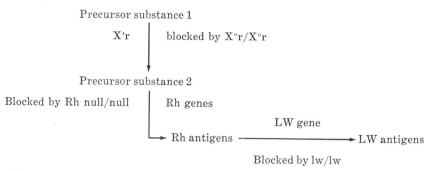

Rare individuals who are homozygous for Rh null will have no detectable Rh antigen or LW antigens, whereas individuals homozygous for the lw gene (lwlw) will lack only the LW antigen and will have a normal complement of Rh antigens.

■ **What is the antigen f (hr) (Rh_6)?**

Antigen f (hr) (Rh_6) is a compound Rh antigen present on the erythrocytes of individuals who have inherited a chromosome that contains both a *c (hr')* and *e (hr'')* gene; e.g., *cDe (R⁰)*, *cde (r)*, *cDᵘe*. This antigen f, sometimes called ce, is detected by anti-f. This antibody is useful in genotyping individuals who have the same phenotype—such as *Rᶻr (CDE/cde)* and *R¹R² CDe/cDE*. Erythrocytes with the former genotype will react with anti-f **(hr)** **(Rh₆)** whereas the latter will not.

■ **Describe the antibodies of the Rh blood group system.**

Naturally occurring antibodies. Naturally occurring antibodies of the Rh blood group system have been described in only isolated instances. The most common naturally occurring antibody in the Rh system is anti-rh'' **(E)**. They are primarily IgM antibodies reacting with saline suspended cells. Weak "naturally occurring" incomplete anti-Rh₀ **(D)** have been recorded. To be classified as a naturally occurring antibody the person so involved must have never been a recipient of blood nor have been pregnant.

Immune antibodies. Immune antibodies to all of the Rh factors (antigens) except Hr₀ (d) have been described. They are found in certain individuals following a blood transfusion or a pregnancy in which they are exposed to a foreign agglutinogen (antigen). Rh₀ (D) is the most potent Rh antigen, followed by hr' (c), rh' (C), rh'' (E), and hr'' (e).

Rh antibodies are generally IgM saline reacting when they first appear following immunization. Subsequently incomplete primarily IgG antibodies develop. They are detectable by the anti-human globulin, enzyme, and high protein methods. They react best at 37° C. Rh antibodies do not fix complement and therefore are not hemolytic.

■ **What is unusual about the Xg blood group system?**

The Xg blood group described first in 1961 is unusual in that it represents the only known blood group system in which the genes are carried on the X chromosome. The gene *Xgᵃ* is responsible for the antigen Xgᵃ which is present in about 89% of females and 66% males. An allele, *Xg*, has been postulated; however, no antibodies to this proposed antigen have been detected. Anti-**Xgᵃ** is detected by the anti-human globulin technique. Females can be of the genotype *XgᵃXgᵃ*, *XgᵃXg*, or *XgXg* whereas males can be either *Xgᵃ* or *Xg*.

■ **What is the practical importance of the I blood group system?**

The antigens of the I blood group system are I and i. The I antigen is a public antigen and adults negative for this antigen are extremely rare. Umbilical cord blood, on the other hand, is only weakly reactive to anti-I. During the first year and a half of life, erythrocytes become more strongly reactive to anti-I and less reactive to anti-i.

Anti-I, a cold agglutinin, is present in very low titers in the serum of most healthy adults. During and following atypical pneumonia caused by *Mycoplasma pneumoniae*, the cold agglutinin titer may increase many fold. High titers of anti-I are also found in those rare individuals ($<0.01\%$) whose erythrocytes are I negative (ii). Certain autoimmune hemolytic anemias present in elderly individuals are caused by the presence of potent auto anti-I. These latter individuals often have malignancies involving the reticuloendothelial system.

There may be considerable difficulty crossmatching blood for an individual with anti-I, as this antibody will react with all red cells including the cells of the patient. It is an IgM immunoglobulin that reacts best with saline suspended erythrocytes at 4° C. Autoabsorption techniques may be required to rid the specimen of this antibody prior to performing the crossmatches. A check for decreased reactivity with cord cells may also be done to help specify the antibody.

■ **Briefly identify and discuss the importance of some of the other blood group systems.**

The human erythrocyte possesses numerous other antigens besides those of the ABO and Rh systems. Two events led to the discovery of the many blood group systems. The first was the widespread utilization of transfusion therapy since the early 1940's. The second was the development of the anti-human globulin test in 1945 by Coombs, Mourant, and Race.

1. MNSs blood group system—1927, Landsteiner and Levine
   Importance: hemolytic disease of the newborn (HDN), transfusion reactions (TR), and paternity
   Incidence: 78% M positive
   72% N positive

2. P blood group system—1927, Landsteiner and Levine
   Importance: TR
   Incidence: 70% P positive

3. Lutheran blood group system—1945, Callendar, Race, and Poykoc
   Importance: HDN, TR
   Incidence: 99.9% Lu^b positive
   8% Lu^a positive

4. Lewis blood group—1946, Mourant
   Importance: TR
   Incidence: 23% Le^a positive
   74% Le^b positive
   4% Le^a negative (Caucasians)
   23% Le^a and Le^b negative (Negroes)

5. Kell blood group system—1946, Coombs, Mourant, and Race
   Importance: HDN, TR
   Incidence: 9% K (Kell) positive
   99.8% k (Cellano) positive
   2% Kp^a (Penny) positive
   99.9% Kp^b (Rautenberg) positive
   0.1% Js^a (Sutter) positive (Caucasians)
   19% Js^a (Sutter) positive (Negroes)
   99% Js^b (Sutter) positive

6. Duffy blood group system—1950, Cutbush, Mollison, and Parkin
   Importance: HDN, TR
   Incidence: 66% Fy^a positive (Caucasians)
   10% Fy^a positive (Negroes)
   83% Fy^b positive (Caucasians)
   23% Fy^b positive (Negroes)
   68% Fy^a and Fy^b negative (Negroes)

7. Kidd blood group system—1951, Allen, Diamond, and Niedziela
   Importance: HDN, TR
   Incidence: 77% Jk^a positive
   73% Jk^b positive
   93% Jk^a positive (Negroes)

8. Diego blood group—1958, Giblett
   Importance: HDN
   Incidence: 100% Di^a negative (Caucasians)
   36% Di^a positive (South American Indians)
   10% Di^a positive (Chinese and Japanese)

9. Auberger blood group—1961, Salmon, Liberge, Andre, Tippett, and Sanger
   Importance: potential HDN and TR; only one example of anti-Au^a has been found
   Incidence: 82% Au positive (Caucasians)

10. Xg blood group system—1962, Mann and associates
    Importance: A sex-linked blood group system with the responsible gene carried on the X chromosome
    Incidence: 89%of female Xg^a positive
    67% of males Xg^a positive

11. Dombrock system—1964, Swanson, Tippett, and Sanger
    Importance: potential TR
    Incidence: 64% Do^a positive

12. Colton blood group system—1967, Heist and associates
    Importance: potential TR

Incidence: 99.7% Co^a positive
                10% Co^b positive

13. Public antigens—other red cell antigens with an incidence greater than 99%: Vel, I, Yt^a, Ge, Sm, Chido, Lan, Gy^a, Gn^a, At^a

14. Private antigens—antigens found only in members of certain families: Levay, Jobbins, Becker, Van, Wr^a, Be^a, Good, Webb, Swann, Bu, Tr^a, Wb, and others

■ **What is the T receptor (antigen)?**

All human red cells contain a latent T antigen that can be activated by enzymes produced by certain bacteria. T-activated cells are agglutinated by anti-**T**, present in all human sera except newborn. These cells are not agglutinated by their own serum. T-activation (Hubner-Thomsen-Friedenreich phenomenon) results in polyagglutinable red cells and difficulty in red cell grouping.

■ **What is the HL-A system?**

The HL-A system is composed of multiple antigens present in various body tissues including the leukocytes and platelets. Antibodies that react with the antigens of this system are responsible for some febrile transfusion reactions and rejection of allografts. The antigens are determined by four genes located on a single pair of chromosomes. Each chromosome of the pair has two independent segregant HL-A subloci (LA or first sublocus and Four or second

Table 6. Alleles associated with the first or LA sublocus and the second or Four sublocus*

LA or first sublocus alleles	*Four or second locus alleles*
HL-A1	HL-A5
HL-A2	HL-A7⟨W22
HL-A3	⟩W27
HL-A9⟨W23	
⟩W24	HL-A8
	HL-A12
	HL-A13
HL-10⟨W25	W5
⟩W26	W10
HL-A11	W14
W29	W15
W30	W16
W31	W17
W32	W18
	W21

*Alleles identified by prefix HL-A have been accepted by the World Health Organization. The prefix W indicates alleles not recognized by the World Health Organization.

sublocus), which are referred to as a haplotype. One haplotype is inherited from each parent and, therefore, individuals possess two LA alleles and two Four alleles, for example, HL-A 1,8/2,7.

The numbers of alleles belonging to the LA or the Four subloci are still increasing and are listed in Table 6.

■ **List some of the criteria for blood donor selection.**

A. Health: exclude potential donors with chronic disease of heart, lungs, kidneys, or liver or history of cancer

B. Age: 17 through 65 years

C. Temperature: must not exceed 99.6° F

D. Hemoglobin or hematocrit:
1. Males—exclude those with less than 13.5 gm hemoglobin/dl or less than 41% hematocrit
2. Females—exclude those with less than 12.5 gm hemoglobin/dl or less than 38% hematocrit

E. Pulse: must be regular and between 50 and 110 beats per minute

F. Blood pressure: must be between 90 and 180 mm Hg systolic and 50 and 100 mm Hg diastolic

G. Pregnancy: exclude those pregnant as well as those pregnant within past 6 months

H. Dental surgery: exclude if less than 72 hours before time of anticipated donation

I. Recipient of blood or blood component: exclude if received less than 6 months before anticipated donation

J. Infectious disease:
1. Viral hepatitis excluded permanently
2. Malaria—donations must be deferred for 3 years after becoming asymptomatic and cessation of therapy
3. Syphilis: exclude if serologic test is positive

K. Immunization: donations are acceptable:
1. 24 hours after immunization with toxoids or killed viral, bacterial, or rickettsial vaccines (e.g., tetanus, diphtheria, influenza, and polio [Salk])
2. 2 weeks after measles, oral polio, mumps, or yellow fever vaccine
3. 2 weeks after an immune smallpox reaction or after the scab has fallen off a primary smallpox reaction
4. 3 months after German measles vaccine
5. 1 year after therapeutic rabies vaccine

    L. Weight: must be greater than 110 pounds for full 450 ml donation.

■ **Describe the collection of blood from a donor.**

The phlebotomist must be trained and under the supervision of a licensed physician, who must be available for consultation during blood collection. A system of numerical identification must be utilized so that it will be possible to relate the donor record, the unit of blood, and the pilot tube. The blood container and the pilot tube must be numerically identified and the pilot tube attached to the collection container, all prior to phlebotomy.

Both arms must be inspected for evidence of recent venipunctures and other lesions. Venipuncture is performed only after adequate preparation of the skin to assure asepsis and a sterile product.

The blood container must be sterile and contain sufficient anticoagulant for the amount of blood to be collected. During collection, the unit must be continually mixed and collected within 7 minutes. This is especially important if components are to be prepared. Following collection, the blood must be promptly refrigerated between 1 and 6° C. Units to be utilized for platelets should not be refrigerated but immediately centrifuged and processed.

Specific instructions for the prevention and treatment of donor reaction must be readily available. Donors must be instructed in possible postphlebotomy reaction such as syncope and should be closely observed for at least 15 minutes prior to leaving the blood bank.

■ **What procedures are performed upon blood that is to be utilized for transfusion purposes?**

The ABO type is determined by (1) testing the red cells with antisera meeting FDA standards and (2) testing the serum for expected antibodies with known A_1 and B red cells. Both results must be in agreement. The Rh_0 (D) type must be determined utilizing anti-**Rh_0** (D) serum meeting requirements of the FDA. Tests designed to detect weak Rh_0 variants (D^u) must be performed on all bloods initially typed as Rh_0 (D) negative. Routine determination of additional Rh factors need not be done.

All donor sera must be tested for the presence of unexpected antibodies using reagent red blood cells meeting FDA standards, using techniques able to demonstrate agglutinating, hemolyzing, and coating antibodies. In addition to the above, all blood must be tested for syphilis by an acceptable serologic test and for the hepatitis B antigen. A positive finding in either case is reason for not utilizing the blood for transfusion purposes.

■ **What procedures are performed on recipient blood prior to transfusion?**

The most important and first step in the preparation of blood for transfusion purposes is to correctly identify the recipient and adequately label the recipient blood sample at the time it is collected. If possible, the potential recipient of blood should be asked to spell his name. This name, along with the hospital and room number, date and hour the specimen was obtained, and initials of the phlebotomist must be placed on a label, which must be firmly affixed to the sample tube before leaving the recipient. An error in recipient identification may be fatal.

The ABO and Rh type are determined on the recipient sample using reagents and methods as described for donor, except testing for Rh_0 variant (D^u) need not be done. Testing with anti-Rh_0 (D) must include an autocontrol (recipient serum–recipient cells) to avoid incorrectly designating an Rh_0 (D) negative recipient as Rh_0 (D) positive. The recipient's serum must also be tested for the presence of unexpected antibodies using reagent blood cells that meet FDA requirements. Blood bank records of previous hospital admissions must be readily available so they may be compared with the results of current testing.

The "major crossmatch" (recipient serum–donor cells) must include a room temperature saline phase with at least a 15-minute incubation period and an anti-human globulin method.

A "minor crossmatch" need not be done, as both the recipient and donor sera are tested for regular and irregular antibodies.

■ **Discuss the proper method of administration of blood and its components.**

The person responsible for the administration of blood obtains a properly labeled unit of blood or blood component from the blood bank. The label attached to the blood must include the recipient's name, hospital and room number, the result of the compatibility tests, the signature of the individual who performed the compatibility tests, and the date performed. A transfusion record must also be provided by the blood bank with each unit to be transfused. This record, a copy of which must be placed on the recipient's chart and a copy sent to the blood bank following completion of the transfusion, must include the following information: recipient's name, hospital or other identification number, results of ABO and Rh testing of both recipient and donor, results of compatibility testing, and signature of person performing them. It should also include space for the signature of the person administering the blood, attesting to the fact that the recipient was properly identified and that the information on the unit label and transfusion record is correct. The record should also provide a space to indicate whether a reaction occurred.

Following the proper identification of the recipient and donor blood, the transfusion should be administered through a sterile transfusion set containing a filter to retain coagulated material and other precipitate that could harm the recipient. Under no circumstances should medication be added to blood.

A responsible individual should be in constant attendance for at least the first 15 minutes of each transfusion, and at regular intervals thereafter.

The rate of transfusion should be determined by the physician. During the first 15 minutes of observation, the rate should not exceed 5 ml/minute. If no adverse reactions are detected, the rate may be increased to 10 ml/minute so that the unit is infused in 45 to 90 minutes. If the cardiac status is in question, or the patient is severely chronically anemic (Hb of 5 gm or less), the rate should not exceed 1 ml/pound/hour and should be given only as red cells.

■ **Discuss hemolytic disease of the newborn; include its pathogenesis.**

Hemolytic disease of the newborn is a disease in which immune destruction and decreased survival of fetal erythrocytes occur because of interaction of these erythrocytes with maternal IgG isoagglutinins that have crossed the placenta. The infant may exhibit anemia, edema, hepatosplenomegaly, hyperbilirubinemia, and, in severe cases, central nervous system damage (kernicterus), even death from heart failure.

Isoimmunization of mothers may occur following transplacental passage of fetal erythrocytes into the maternal circulation during the last trimester of pregnancy and at the time of separation of the placenta following delivery. Sensitization may also follow blood transfusion.

Hemolytic disease of the newborn can result from fetomaternal incompatibilities in the Rh, ABO, Kell, Duffy, and other blood group systems. The former two are the most common, and Rh_0 (D) hemolytic disease is generally the severest. ABO hemolytic disease of the newborn occurs almost exclusively in group A or B infants born to group O mothers, while Rh hemolytic disease occurs most commonly in Rh_0 (D) positive infants born to sensitized Rh_0 (D) negative mothers.

■ **Describe prenatal evaluation for hemolytic disease of the newborn.**

There are three avenues available for the correct prenatal assessment of the severity of possible hemolytic disease of the newborn: (1) history of the fate of previous infants, (2) erythrocyte antigen and serum antibody studies, and (3) amniotic fluid studies. No one avenue is adequate and all three may be necessary to correctly evaluate the individual situation. The following laboratory studies are suggested for proper evaluation of this problem.

A. At 6 weeks gestational age or first prenatal visit:
   1. ABO and Rh type to include D^u of all mothers
   2. Mother's serum screened for irregular isoagglutinins using reagent red cells
   3. Identify irregular isoagglutinins, if any are detected, using panel of reagent red cells
   4. If mother is Rh_0 (D) negative, determine father's ABO type and probable Rh genotype
   5. Freeze and save mother's serum for future re-titer or reference
B. At 24 to 28 weeks gestation:
   1. Rescreen mother's serum for irregular isoagglutinins
   2. If irregular isoagglutinins are present, identify and titer in parallel with previous serum samples
C. At 22 to 32 weeks gestational age in women with demonstrable antibodies:
   1. Amniocentesis for spectrophotometric analysis of amniotic fluid (a) for baseline studies, (b) to detect severely involved infants for whom delivery at 32 to 37 weeks or intrauterine transfusion could offer a chance for survival
   2. Determine ABO type of the amniotic fluid of secretor infants by hemagglutination inhibition
   3. Identify red cells recovered from amniotic fluid by ABO type, Rh type, and direct anti-human globulin test
D. At 24 to 36 weeks gestational age:

    1. Repeat amniocentesis at 2-week intervals to evaluate need for intrauterine transfusion or premature delivery

E. At 34 to 35 weeks gestational age:
    1. Rescreen mother's serum for irregular isoagglutinins; especially important in Rh_0 (D) negative mothers

F. Prior to delivery of mother with irregular isoagglutinins:
    1. The blood bank should be notified of impending delivery as soon as possible so that blood may be immediately available at delivery for exchange transfusion if indicated

■ **Discuss prevention of maternal Rh_0 (D) sensitization.**

Levine recognized that Rh_0 (D) sensitization is more common in ABO compatible than in incompatible matings. Subsequent observations and studies revealed that Rh_0 (D) sensitization is prevented if IgG anti-Rh_0 (D) is administered to the mother within 72 hours of delivery of a Rh_0 (D) positive child, or following miscarriage or therapeutic abortion. This passive immunization is 98 to 99.5% effective in preventing sensitization to Rh_0 (D).

The following should be performed for maximum benefit from anti-Rh_0 (D) immunoglobulin therapy.

    1. Determine Rh_0 (D) type (including D^u) on all expectant mothers.

    2. Screen all Rh_0 (D) negative mothers for irregular isoagglutinins.

    3. Determine Rh_0 (D) type (including D^u) on cord blood from babies of Rh_0 (D) negative mothers.

    4. Perform direct anti-human globulin test on cord blood.

The mother is a candidate for anti-Rh_0 (D) immunoglobulin therapy if the following criteria are met: (a) she is Rh_0 (D) negative and D^u negative; (b) she is not immunized to the Rh_0 (D) factor, as determined following delivery; (c) the baby is Rh_0 (D) positive or D^u positive; and (d) the baby has a negative direct anti-human globulin test. The mother is still a candidate if the baby has a positive direct anti-human globulin test because of an antibody other than anti-Rh_0 (D).

A dose of 1 ml (300 μg) of anti-Rh_0 (D) immunoglobulin is given intramuscularly to the mother following a compatible minor crossmatch. An incompatible crossmatch and/or positive maternal D^u in a mother previously determined to be Rh_0 (D) and D^u negative may indicate a massive transplacental hemorrhage, necessitating more than a 1 ml dose. The magnitude of the fetal-maternal hemorrhage may be estimated by identifying fetal red cells in the maternal blood utilizing the Kleihauer acid elution test. Fetal cells contain fetal hemoglobin, which resists acid elution.

Therapy should also be given to Rh_0 (D) negative women following miscarriage or therapeutic abortion.

- **Discuss amniocentesis as a tool in monitoring suspected hemolytic disease of the newborn.**

In 1953 Bevis first suggested that examination of amniotic fluid could give valuable information in the evaluation of an unborn child with potential hemolytic disease of the newborn. This concept was further expanded by Liley and others in the early 1960's. After the amniotic fluid is obtained, it must be protected from light and clarified by centrifugation. The fluid is then scanned in a narrow band spectrophotometer to determine the presence of a 450 nm absorption peak, which represents breakdown products of hemoglobin. A normal amniotic fluid scan has no significant 450 nm peak, while fluid from a pregnancy with hemolytic disease has an absorption peak with a 450 nm maximum.

The severity of the hemolytic disease can be assessed by the net density of the 450 nm peak. Liley plotted optical density versus gestational age and developed three zones of involvment. Zone 1 peaks indicate mild or no involvement. Zone 2 peaks suggest moderate involvement requiring careful observation and follow-up. Zone 3 peaks suggest severe disease, usually requiring intrauterine transfusions or immediate delivery of the child. Amniotic fluid studies are also utilized to determine fetal maturity, sex, fetal blood groups, and chromosomal and biochemical abnormalities.

- **Discuss selection of blood for a newborn with hemolytic disease of the newborn.**

Blood selected for transfusion therapy of the newborn must be compatible with serum from the mother. Subsequent transfusions must be compatible with serum of both the mother and the baby. Antibodies present in the newborn's serum are present in the maternal serum in invariably greater quantities. Utilization of maternal serum also enables the blood bank to obtain and crossmatch blood for the baby prior to delivery.

It is preferable to use blood that is less than 3 but no more than 5 days old. An attempt should be made to utilize, if possible, blood that is of the same ABO group as the baby and negative for the offending antigen. When the mother is group O, group O blood must be used. In the latter situation, if the child is other than group O, red cells or hemolysin free whole blood should be given.

■ **What are the indications for transfusion therapy?**

Blood and blood component therapy can be life-saving and at other times a valuable therapeutic procedure. However, because of hidden dangers that may be present, a prescription for blood or component therapy should be made only with justifiable indication. Component rather than whole blood therapy should be utilized so that more than one patient may be treated with a single donation. Following are the major indications.

1. To maintain blood volume and treat hypovolemic shock. Severe massive, acute blood loss is probably the only indication for whole blood therapy.
2. To improve oxygen-carrying capacity. This is best treated with red blood cells rather than whole blood.
3. To replace platelets and other coagulation factors that are deficient in persons with hemorrhagic disorders.
4. Exchange transfusion to treat newborns with hemolytic disease and persons with hepatic coma.

■ **What are red blood cells?**

Red blood cells are prepared from whole blood by removing two-thirds of the plasma-anticoagulant solution so that the hematocrit is about 60 to 70%. This separation is accomplished by sedimentation or centrifugation. If separation is done in a closed system, the red cells may be transfused up to 21 days from the date of collection.

Red blood cells should be utilized whenever the indication is to improve oxygen-carrying capacity. In addition to being an efficient method of achieving this, red cells reduce the possibility of circulatory overload. They also contain less sodium, acid, potassium, and ammonia than whole blood and are less likely to aggravate cardiac, renal, and hepatic failures when they exist.

■ **What is the indication for platelet concentrate therapy?**

Platelet concentrates are administered to individuals bleeding as a result of thrombocytopenia.

Platelets are obtained from whole blood by differential centrifugation and can be used only for 72 hours from the time of collection.

■ **Discuss cryoprecipitate.**

Cryoprecipitate contains primarily factor VIII and some fibrinogen. It is prepared by thawing fresh frozen plasma between 2 and 6° C. Following centrifugation the supernatant plasma is removed and the cryoprecipitate that remains is refrozen. When needed for transfusion, it is thawed at 37° C and dissolved in 10 ml of saline. Each unit of cryoprecipitate contains about 80 to 120 units of factor VIII. A unit of factor VIII is defined as the factor VIII activity in 1 ml of fresh normal plasma.

Cryoprecipitate is used in the treatment of hemorrhage occurring in hemophilia. It has also been used in the treatment of hypofibrinogenemia. Superconcentrates of factor VIII containing up to 1,000 units per container are available commercially.

■ **Discuss frozen red blood cells.**

The shelf-life of red blood cells can be extended almost indefinitely by freezing and storing at ultralow temperatures in the presence of a cryoprotective agent such as glycerol. At the time of use the cells must be thawed and washed to remove the glycerol, and transfused within 24 hours. Presently, because of cost, the use of frozen red blood cells is limited, but as technology advances freezing will probably become the prime method of storage. Massachusetts General Hospital, Boston, and Cook County Hospital, Chicago, are now almost exclusively using frozen red cells.

■ **What are some of the hazards of transfusion therapy?**

Adverse reactions can be divided into immediate and delayed types. A reaction is any unfavorable symptom experienced by the recipient. An immediate reaction occurs within minutes or hours following start of a transfusion, whereas a delayed reaction occurs days or weeks following a transfusion.

A. Immediate reactions
   1. Hemolytic transfusion reactions
     a. Hemolysis related to blood group incompatibility
     b. Hemolysis related to faulty administration of blood through 5% dextrose or 5% dextrose in 0.25% saline
   2. Reactions secondary to administration of bacterially contaminated blood
   3. Circulatory overload reactions
   4. Pyrogenic reactions
     a. Exogenous pyrogens—bacterial
     b. Endogenous pyrogens—caused by disease state of recipient

  c. Leukoagglutinins—common in females who have had multiple pregnancies

  d. Platelet agglutinins

 5. Allergic reactions—hives, bronchospasm, and/or generalized anaphylaxis may occur following administration of blood or plasma containing a protein component to which the recipient is sensitive; serious anaphylactic transfusion reactions occur in individuals with IgA deficiency who have been immunized to IgA

 6. Hemorrhagic diathesis following massive transfusions

 7. Air embolism—rare since widespread usage of plastic bags

 8. Citrate toxicity (rare) may result in hypocalcemia in individuals with impaired liver function

B. Delayed reactions

 1. Transmission of disease

  a. Viral hepatitis

  b. Syphilis

  c. Malaria

  d. Chagas' disease

  e. Brucellosis

 2. Isosensitization—may prevent or make difficult transfusion therapy in the future, as well as placing in jeopardy the fate of future children of women of childbearing age

 3. Transfusional siderosis—follows transfusion of large quantities of blood over prolonged periods (Remember: each unit of blood contains 250 mg of iron.)

■ **Why is CPD anticoagulation and preservation of blood superior to that of ACD?**

Until recently, blood obtained for transfusion purposes was drawn almost exclusively into acid-citrate-dextrose (ACD) solution. This solution is an anticoagulant and preservative allowing a shelf-life of 21 days, which is the maximum storage time that 70% of the red cells will survive 24 hours in a recipient when transfused.

The oxygen dissociation curve of blood preserved in ACD solution shifts significantly to the left ($\downarrow P_{50}$). Therefore, ACD blood has a decreased ability to release oxygen to the tissues, because the affinity of hemoglobin for oxygen is increased.

The concentration of the red cell 2,3-diphosphoglycerate (2,3-DPG) is inversely proportional to the affinity of hemoglobin for oxygen. During storage of blood in ACD the concentration of red cell 2,3-DPG decreases and the affinity of hemoglobin for oxygen is increased.

Studies of blood drawn in citrate-phosphate-dextrose (CPD) have shown that the 24-hour 70% red cell survival is maintained for 28 days following collection. More important, blood collected in CPD retains a higher 2,3-DPG concentration for a longer period of time, which results in a lesser shift to the left in the oxygen dissociation curve. Thus hemoglobin will more readily release oxygen to the tissues.

The above are a few reasons why the anticoagulant-preservative of choice is CPD. Major blood banks throughout the country have changed to this anticoagulant. The FDA has licensed CPD blood for only a 21-day "out date," similar to that for ACD blood. Rejuvenating solutions containing substances such as pyruvate, inosine, adenine, and phosphate may in the future be utilized to improve the 24-hour posttransfusion survival of red cells.

CHAPTER 4

Urinology

OPAL KELLY

■ **What is pH?**

pH is a measurement of free hydrogen (H+) ions in the urine. It reflects the ability of the kidney to maintain normal H+ ion concentration in the plasma and extracellular fluid (ECF). Urine pH will range from 4.5 to 8.0. Knowledge of pH in a fresh urine specimen may be of assistance in evaluating metabolic disorders. Urine is very acid in diabetic ketoacidosis. In renal tubular acidosis (RTA) the urine is persistently neutral to alkaline. In potassium deficiency the pH tends to rise. In some urinary tract infections, in which a "urea-splitting" organism is present, an alkaline urine is formed.

■ **What are the ketone bodies?**

The ketone bodies are beta hydroxybutyric acid, acetoacetic acid, and acetone. Beta hydroxybutyric acid and acetoacetic acid decompose into acetone on standing. Ketonuria occurs most frequently in uncontrolled diabetes mellitus. It may also occur in acute febrile and toxic states, vomiting, and following anesthesia, and is probably caused by increased catabolism and limited food intake.

■ **Why is a test for sugar done?**

Routine testing for sugar may be done using a dipstick, testing only for glucose. The urine should be at room temperature. Using an alkaline copper sulfate, one may test for all reducing substances. Sugars that reduce copper sulfate to cuprous oxide are glucose, lactose, galactose, fructose, and pentose. These sugars may be identified by thin layer chromatography.

Glucose in the urine with a high blood sugar indicates diabetes mellitus. Glucose in the urine with a normal blood sugar indicates renal glycosuria.

■ **When is occult blood found?**

The occult blood test may be positive when either large numbers of RBC's (hematuria) or hemoglobin (hemoglobinuria) is present. Hemoglobinuria may be caused by intravascular hemolysis, transfusion reaction, or lysis of cells from standing in very dilute urine.

■ **When may proteinuria occur?**

Proteinuria may occur as the result of any of the following: (1) disruption of normal glomerular capillary permeability such as occurs through antigen-antibody complement deposition, as in acute post-streptococcal glomerulonephritis or systemic lupus erythematosus (SLE) with renal involvement; (2) tubular proteinuria—there is an increased excretion of plasma proteins in the presence of a normal glomerulus; the small molecular size of the Bence Jones protein is readily filtered and excreted in the urine; or (3) the irritative effect of infection may result in increased exudation of plasma proteins into the urine; however, this amounts to only a few hundred mg per day.

■ **What is orthostatic proteinuria?**

It is an abnormal protein excretion only in the upright position. There may be as much as 1,000 mg per 24 hours. When the individual is at rest the abnormal protein completely disappears. The precise mechanism is unknown but is considered to be a nonglomerular type of proteinuria and thus not pathologic.

■ **When cloudy urines are received, how can they be cleared?**

When urine stands and cools below body temperature, crystals may precipitate and should be dissolved before centrifuging. In acid urine, urates precipitate causing a pink cloud, "brick dust," and can be dissolved by warming the urine to 60° C. In alkaline urine, phosphates form a white cloud and can be dissolved by the addition of a few drops of 5% acetic acid. This will not destroy cells or casts. Cells and casts will be obscured by the amorphous material.

■ **What is specific gravity?**

Specific gravity compares the weight of a liquid with the weight of distilled H_2O and measures the relative amount of solids in the urine. There are technical limitations in using the urinometer. Temperature affects the specific gravity. The urinometer should be standardized daily in distilled water at room temperature. Protein and glucose raise specific gravity. In diabetics the glucose correction may be necessary when doing a concentration test.

■ **What is osmolality?**

Osmolality is the measurement of osmotically active particles. The freezing depression point (FDP) is measured and converted to osmotic pressure. The FDP is the temperature at which a solute changes from a liquid to a solid state. One milliosmol will lower the freezing point $-0.00186°$ C.

■ **What is concentration and dilution?**

It describes the degree to which the nephron changes the solute density above or below that of the plasma ultrafiltrate before it is excreted as urine.

■ **After 12 hours of fluid restriction, what concentration does normal urine reach?**

After fluids have been restriced for 12 to 16 hours, usually over the night hours, a specific gravity of at least 1.025 should be attained and a urine osmolality greater than 800 mOsm.

■ **Why is the microscopic examination of the urine essential?**

The microscopic examination may be called "a liquid biopsy of the kidney." There may be a direct disease relationship to the findings in the urine sediment.

■ **What are casts?**

Casts are molds of the tubule and occur because of "gelling" of the protein. The protein is Tamm-Horsfal, which is apparently secreted by the cells lining the distal part of the nephron. It is readily precipitated in a urine of low pH and specific gravity. Casts may be absent in chronic renal disease even though proteinuria is significant because the capacity to form acid and concentrated urine has been lost.

■ **Can the width of a cast be an indication of the severity of renal disease?**

Casts are thought to form in the distal or collecting tubule. Broad casts are probably formed in the collecting tubules. Large numbers of broad casts indicate widespread stasis in the nephron.

■ **How is the width of a cast judged?**

A narrow cast is 1 to 2 RBC's in width; a medium cast is 3 to 4 RBC's in width; and the broad cast is greater than 5 RBC's in width.

■ **What are hyaline casts?**

Hyaline casts are precipitated protein without formed elements. In small numbers they are not clinically significant but are associated with proteinuria and therefore are seen in almost every clinical situation.

■ **What are cell casts?**

Epithelial cell casts are composed largely of desquamated epithelial cells as a result of intrinsic renal disease. These casts may be difficult to distinguish from WBC casts unless the structure is intact. In WBC casts, the cells have become enmeshed in the protein matrix. They may be found in acute pyelonephritis or noninflammatory diseases such as acute glomerulonephritis and SLE. The casts should be carefully distinguished from clumped WBC's.

In RBC casts, the RBC's have become enmeshed in the protein matrix. The cast is usually red-orange in color. The individual cells may be difficult to identify because they are so tightly packed. The RBC cast is indicative of glomerulitis.

■ **What are granular casts?**

Granular casts are probably the result of casts "lying in the tubule" and have degenerated from epithelial cells, WBC or RBC casts, and protein. Some cellular material may still be evident. They may be classed as coarse or fine.

■ **What are fatty casts?**

Casts containing fat droplets are called "fatty casts." They are found with oval fat bodies (OFB), free fat droplets, and heavy proteinuria and are associated with the nephrotic syndrome.

■ **What is the nephrotic syndrome?**

The nephrotic syndrome is characterized by edema, proteinuria 3 to 4+ qualitatively and greater than 3.5 gm quantitatively, hypoalbuminemia, and hyperlipemia. In the microscopic may be found the fatty cast, OFB, free fat droplets, and hyaline and granular casts. RBC's and tubular epithelial cells are variable. RBC casts are rarely found. Depending on etiology, renal function may not be markedly impaired.

Some of the diseases in which the nephrotic syndrome may occur are glomerulonephritis, diabetic glomerulosclerosis, systemic lupus erythematosus, and occasionally as the result of allergins, insect bites, and drugs.

■ **What are some diseases in which RBC's, RBC casts, and protein occur?**

When RBC casts and heavy protein are found, the disease is

usually glomerular: (1) acute poststreptococcal glomerulonephritis; (2) glomerulitis associated with diseases such as SLE, Good-
pasture's syndrome, Henoch-Schöenlein purpura, and thrombotic
thrombocytopenic purpura; or (3) malignant nephrosclerosis.
RBC's and RBC casts without heavy proteinuria may also be found
in glomerulonephritis, subacute bacterial endocarditis (SBE), and
hereditary nephritis.

■ **When would you find RBC's with minimal proteinuria?**

Proteinuria is minimal with RBC's when there is a focal urinary
tract disease: (1) tumor, (2) infection, (3) stone, (4) trauma,
(5) polycystic kidney disease, (6) clotting disorders, and (7)
sickle cell trait.

■ **What is glomerular filtrate?**

The glomerular filtrate is essentially protein free and free of
all cells. It is composed of water and dissolved solids such as electrolytes, amino acids, urea, and all substances unbound to protein
and capable of being in solution.

■ **What properties must a substance have to be suitable for use in
measurement of the glomerular filtration rate (GFR)?**

To adequately measure GFR, a substance must be freely filtered
and remain fairly constant in transit through the nephron, being
neither secreted, reabsorbed, nor diffused. Inulin completely satis-
fies this requirement.

■ **What is clearance?**

Clearance is the volume of blood plasma completely cleared of
a substance, by renal excretion, in 1 minute.

$$C = \frac{UV}{P}$$

C = Clearance of a substance
U = Urine concentration of a substance
V = Volume of urine collected over a given period of time
P = Mean plasma concentration of a substance during the
time of urine formation

■ **What is creatinine clearance (C_{cr})?**

Creatinine is a byproduct of protein metabolism and is produced at a constant rate depending upon the muscle mass of the
individual. Creatinine is freely filtered by the glomerulus and is
considered to be neither secreted nor reabsorbed. Urine should
be collected over long periods of time. Twenty-four hours is the
best period of time to minimize collection error. Normal C_{cr} is
90-140 ml/minute with an average of 120 ml/minute/M^2, or 100
to 180 L/24 hours/1.73 M^2.

■ **Why is creatinine clearance preferred to urea clearance?**

Urea clearance has been the most commonly used test to estimate GFR because urea is exclusively excreted by the kidney, although factors other than GFR affect urea. Low urine flow results in increased urea absorption. The optimum urine flow should be greater than 2 ml/minute. The daily production of urea is highly variable and depends partly on protein intake. Starvation will result in decreased BUN levels. GI bleeding and tissue catabolism such as fever will cause increased BUN levels. Thus, using urea clearance as an index of GFR is misleading.

■ **What are some of the things necessary for an accurate renal clearance?**

To assure accuracy of renal clearance, the total urine must be collected during a precise period of time. If short clearance periods are used, such as 1 or 2 hours, a brisk urine flow should be established to ensure spontaneous voiding and complete emptying of the bladder. This can be achieved with adequate hydration. If fluids must be restricted because of impaired renal function, longer clearance periods should be used.

■ **When will bilirubin be found?**

Bilirubin is the breakdown product of hemoglobin. It is found in the urine of patients with obstructive jaundice or liver damage caused by exposure to toxins or ingestion of certain drugs. It may appear in the urine of patients with hepatitis before clinical jaundice appears.

■ **When will urobilinogen appear in the urine?**

Urobilinogen is the product of bilirubin oxidation and will be increased in the urine when there is hemolysis of RBC's. It may be elevated in liver disease because the liver cells are not able to reabsorb or reexcrete circulating urobilinogen. It may be absent in the urine when there is complete obstruction of the bile duct. The qualitative test must be performed on fresh urine.

■ **Identify some of the colors of urine.**

Straw, pale, almost watery appearing urine usually indicates a low specific gravity. Yellow is the normal color of urine and indicates a specific gravity of 1.012 to 1.019 with an output of 1 to 1.5 L/day. Amber indicates a concentrated urine, the volume usually under 1 L/day. Some of the abnormal pigments are: brownish yellow or brownish green, which indicates bile; red to red brown, hemoglobinuria; red brown with brown pigmented casts in the sediment, myoglobin; dark brown, methemoglobin. Some foods and drugs will also pigment the urine.

■ **What is an Addis count?**

An Addis count is accurately timed urine with quantitative enumeration of RBC's and WBC's and casts. A precise amount of urine is centrifuged for an exact length of time and then counted on a counting chamber. It is usually collected over night hours after restriction of fluids the day of the test. Twelve hours is the accepted length of time but may be shortened to 6 or 9 hours. The urine should be preserved with formalin. The pH should be low and the concentration high.

■ **What are kidney stones?**

Kidney stones are composed of a mucoprotein matrix, inorganic and organic crystals. The most common stone is the calcium oxalate stone and usually occurs in a sterile urine. There is a familial, probably a genetic predisposition to form calcium oxalate stones. They may also result from hyperparathyroidism, renal tubular acidosis, and idiopathic hypercalcuria. Other types of stones are uric acid, sometimes found in patients with gout and sometimes caused by increased excretion of urates. Magnesium ammonium phosphate stones reflect chronic urinary tract infection with "urea splitting" organisms.

Cystine stones are always associated with patients who have a genetic defect in tubular transport and reabsorption of dibasic amino acids, cystine, lysine, arginine, and ornithine. Stone formation is probably the result of reduced urine volume and increased excretion of calcium, oxalate, uric acid, or ammonia (phosphate), or changes conducive to stone formation at normal concentration of crystalloids, pH particularly. At the time stones are being passed there may be small amounts of protein and hematuria, gross to microscopic. With magnesium ammonium phosphate stones the urine is the same as that of urinary tract infection.

CHAPTER 5

Radiochemistry

RAYMOND ZASTROW

■ **What is a radionuclide?**

A nuclide is any atomic nucleus and its orbital electrons. A radionuclide is a nuclide that emits radioactivity as it forms another nuclide.

■ **What is an isotope?**

An isotope is one or more stable or unstable forms of the same element having the same atomic number. They have the same chemical properties but vary as to radioactive properties.

■ **What types of radiation are useful in radiochemistry?**

There are two basic types of radiation—particle emission and electromagnetic emission.

■ **Explain particle emission.**

During atomic rearrangement (disintegration), depending upon the element involved, a variety of atomic subparticles may be emitted. These include electrons from the atomic orbital rings or nuclear derivatives such as alpha particles, beta particles, and positrons.

■ **What is an alpha particle?**

It is a helium nucleus stripped of its orbital ring of electrons. Since it consists of two protons and two neutrons, it has a positive charge and a mass of 4. Because of this heavy mass, as compared to electrons, beta particles, and positrons, its speed is slow, penetration of tissues is short (measured in micra), and it thus remains in contact with local tissue molecules for a comparatively long time. This contact combined with the 2+ charge of the double protons leads to a high probability of interaction with tissue molecules, resulting in their rearrangement. This rearrangement is called ionization.

■ **What are electrons?**

Electrons are high-speed, negatively charged particles arranged in orbital rings about a nucleus. Their weight is 1/1,840 that of a neutron. Because of the low weight and high speed, the chance for contact with individual tissue items is lessened and the specific ionization is a fraction of that of the alpha particles. The tissue penetration, however, is deeper (measured in millimeters).

■ **What is a beta particle, or negatron?**

Beta particles are negatively charged particles arising from the nucleus secondary to nuclear rearrangement. Their charge, weight, speed, penetration, and specific ionization are identical to those of the electron.

■ **What is a positron?**

Positrons are also nuclear derivatives emitted during disintegration. They carry a positive charge but in all other respects are similar to beta particles.

■ **What are the types of electromagnetic radiation?**

The electromagnetic spectrum includes visible light, radiowaves, microwaves, and so on. The highest frequency electromagnetic spectra are of interest to radiochemistry—the gamma photons and x-ray photons.

■ **What are gamma photons?**

Gamma photons are high-energy, high-frequency electromagnetic forces derived during nuclear rearrangement. They travel at the speed of light and thus have high peneration and low specific ionization.

■ **How do x-rays differ from gamma photons?**

X-rays are derived during orbital electron rearrangements. They also travel at the speed of light and in other respects are similar to gamma photons.

■ **What does the M in technetium-99M mean?**

The suffix M indicates a metastable state. It indicates an atom undergoing decay but yet retaining its energy. Technetium (Tc) is a daughter nuclide of molybdenum-99. Its intermediate state is Tc-99M which has a 6-hour half-life.

■ **What is physical half-life (T½)?**

It is the time required for a radionuclide to decay to one-half the number of original atoms. For example, 1 millicurie of a radionuclide will decay to half a millicurie (500 microcuries) in one half-life.

■ **What is a curie?**

It is a unit of activity defined as 3.7×10^{10} disintegrations per second.

■ **What is a millicurie?**

A millicurie is 10^{-3} curies.

■ **What is a microcurie?**

A microcurie is 10^{-6} curies.

■ **What is effective half-life?**

It is the physical half-life combined with the rate of biologic degradation or biologic half-life.

■ **What is specific activity?**

It is the concentration of radioactive material and is usually expressed as millicuries per gram.

■ **What is shielding?**

Various materials may be used to block the energy photons so that they do not strike the technologist or adjacent instrumentation. The thickness required to reduce the amount of radiation on the side opposite the shield is dependent upon the density of the material used.

■ **What is the half value layer?**

It is the thickness of any given shielding material that will reduce the radioactivity on the opposite side from the source by half.

■ **What is a collimator?**

It is a perforated shield used to protect the detector instrument head from extraneous energy photons while acting to direct the specific detection of a given photon source.

■ **What is the inverse square law?**

Radiation exposure and detection levels decrease with the square of the distance from the source. If the distance between the source and the detector head is doubled, the amount of radiation detected is reduced to one-fourth that of the original.

■ **What are the cardinal principles of radiation safety?**

Shielding, distance, physical half-life, good housekeeping, and responsible record keeping. Housekeeping includes correct waste disposal and placarding of radioactive areas. Good record keeping includes the use of film badges, dosimeters, monitoring of the laboratory area, waste disposal records, and adherence to local and federal laws.

■ **What is a RAD?**

The RAD is radiation absorbed dose, the amount of radiation energy absorbed by a given biologic structure. It is used clinically to describe the amount of exposure to a given organ or organs of interest.

■ **What is a roentgen?**

A roentgen is a measure of gamma or x-ray radiation quantity as measured in air. It is used as the amount of exposure dose produced by a source.

■ **What is REM?**

REM is roentgen equivalent man. It is the unit of human absorbed dose. It is used as the exposure value for monitoring devices, as well as for the values for the recommended maximum permissible dose.

■ **What is a crystal scintillation counter?**

It is a thallium activated sodium iodide crystal coupled to a photomultiplier tube. As energy photons enter the crystal and interact with the crystal molecules, minute flashes of light occur. These are detected and magnified by an electronic photomultiplier tube. The resultant electrical energy is amplified and proportionately counted.

■ **What is a liquid scintillation system?**

It is a detector system which measures the beta-producing radiation of a radionuclide dissolved in a liquid scintillation fluid.

■ **Describe a pulse height analyzer.**

Each radionuclide has a distinct energy spectrum. By electronic discrimination, either or both of the lower or higher energy ranges may be rejected, and a given radionuclide energy peak can be maximized for counting without interference by background counts or other radiation sources. The area between this lower threshold and upper threshold is called the "window."

■ **Describe a nuclide generator or "cow."**

It consists of a shielded container in which there is a long-lived parent radionuclide that produces a short-lived daughter nuclide. This short-lived nuclide can be separated and used as needed. An example is molybdenum-99, which produces technetium-99M, having a 6-hour half-life. The technetium can be eluted from the parent molybdenum and used as needed.

■ **Describe the principle of competitive binding.**

Given the stoichiometric reversible reaction such as $Y + Z \leftrightarrows YZ$, the addition of more molecules of Y will result in a proportioned distribution of these new molecules of Y in the end product, YZ. This proportion of distribution is directly related to the concentration of YZ. That is, the greater the concentration of YZ, the more original Y molecules displaced by the new Y! $Y + Y* + Z \leftrightarrows YZ + Y*Z$. If these new molecules of Y can be identified with a radioactive label, and if the parent substance can be separated from the substrate, a value of displacement can be determined. By using a range of standards of YZ, a curve of concentration may be drawn and the concentration of the original substance can be determined.

■ **What is the principle of radioimmunoassay?**

Radioimmunoassay is a saturation and displacement analysis not unlike competitive binding, but using the antigen-antibody reaction rather than the binding protein as the receptor site. Antibody does not discriminate between labeled and unlabeled antigen. Hence, the addition of labeled antigen to a serum having an unknown amount of unlabeled antigen followed by a specific antibody will result in proportional distribution of labeled and unlabeled antigen bound to this antibody. If the amount of original unlabeled antigen is small, i.e., if the patient's serum level is low, proportionately greater amounts of labeled antigen will be bound to antibody and less unlabeled antigen will be free in the reaction mixture. The ratio of this bound to free radioactively detectable antigen will be relatively high. If the patient's serum level is high, the ratio of bound over free radioactive antigen will be relatively smaller. Hence, by drawing a standard curve using increasingly known concentrations of purified antigen, this ratio of bound to free radionuclide can be expressed as a known value.

■ **What is the T3 test?**

Triiodothyronine, T3, is a physiologic precursor to thyroxine, T4. Thyroxine binding globulin (TBG) preferentially binds T4 before it binds T3. In the hyperthyroid state, the TBG is saturated with T4 and any exogenous radioactive T3 incubated with TBG will not be bound. In hypothyroid conditions the TBG will take up the radioactive T3 since binding sites are available. After incubation, the unbound T3 is absorbed and counted. In hyperthyroidism, since there is more available unbound T3, the value obtained will be above the normal range. In hypothyroidism, the value obtained will be below the normal range. When the TBG itself is elevated, especially by pregnancy and birth control medication, the number of binding sites is increased, allowing for increased absorption of radioactive T3 and less residual available for counting. This produces a spurious low count resembling hypothyroidism.

■ **What is the T4 test?**

Thyroxine (T4) is released from the patient's thyroid binding globulin (TBG) by denaturation. This released T4 is incubated with exogenous TBG whose own T4 is labeled with radioactive iodine. In the principle of competitive binding, the original released T4 competes with the labeled T4. The amount of release of the labeled T4 is proportional to the number of original molecules of T4 in the patient. Physical separation extracts the unbound T4. Increased patient thyroxine results in the high release of radioactive counts in the extract and corresponds to hyperthyroidism. A low residual radioactive count indicates the low T4 found in hypothyroidism. The specific assay value can be determined by forming a standard curve using purified thyroxine.

Increased TBG, as seen in pregnancy and contraceptive medication, results in spurious high counts and resembles hyperthyroidism.

■ **What is the T7 test value?**

It is a mathematical formulation using the T3 and T4 values in order to compensate for the high T4 and low T3 in pregnancy and contraceptive medication.

■ **What is the ETR?**

The effective thyroxine ratio (ETR) is a single in vitro procedure that considers the thyroid binding globulin and total serum T4. It combines the competitive binding procedure of the T4 determination with a TBG absorption method analagous to the T3 procedure. It is unaffected by pregnancy or contraceptive medication.

■ **Describe the radioactive iodine uptake.**

The patient receives an oral dose of radioactive iodine. The number of radioactive counts taken over the neck is compared at a timed interval to the number of counts present in a standard geometric form containing an identical dose. The percent uptake is below normal in hypothyroidism or in previous high intake of iodine or x-ray dyes. The uptake is elevated in hyperthyroidism.

■ **Describe the principle of radioactive blood volume determination.**

A known amount of radioactive material is injected intravenously. A similar amount of radioactivity is diluted as a standard pool. After dilution in the patient, a blood sample is drawn and compared to an equivalent sample from the standard pool. The total circulating blood volume can then be mathematically extrapolated.

■ **What radionuclides may be used in determining blood volume?**

Many may be used. However, the radioactive iodinated serum albumin (RISA) labeled with ^{125}I is the most commonly used material.

■ **Can chromium 51 (^{51}Cr) be used for the blood volume?**

Yes. ^{51}Cr labels the red cell. If washed labeled red cells are injected and recovered after equilibration in the patient, comparison to a pool standard and the use of the hematocrit can determine total blood volume.

■ **What is the ^{51}Cr red cell survival?**

^{51}Cr labeled red cells are injected and sampled periodically over 2 to 3 weeks. The loss of radioactivity is compared to the known standard value curve. Rapid loss indicates bleeding or hemolysis.

■ **Describe the Schilling test.**

It is a test for the absorption of vitamin B_{12}. An oral dose of vitamin B_{12} labeled with radioactive cobalt is administered, followed by the collection of a 24-hour urine specimen. If there is reduced intestinal absorption of vitamin B_{12} or lack of gastric intrinsic factor, a small amount of radioactive vitamin B_{12} is recovered in the urine. By repeating the test with the addition of oral intrinsic factor (desiccated hog stomach), the patient whose absorption defect is a lack of his own intrinsic factor, such as in pernicious anemia, will demonstrate more normal recovery of the radioactive material.

■ **Describe the plasma-iron clearance.**

^{59}Fe is injected into the patient. Blood samples are drawn at frequent timed intervals for 2 hours. The time of disappearance of the radio-iron to half of the original is noted. This time is shortened in active marrow turnover, such as iron deficiency or hemolytic anemia.

■ **Describe the plasma-iron turnover rate.**

Using the plasma-iron clearance, the total serum iron, and the total plasma volume, the rate of iron turnover can be determined by formula. This turnover value is increased in active marrow turnover conditions, such as iron deficiency and hemolytic anemia.

■ **Describe red cell utilization.**

Using the same radioactive iron as that given for the plasma-iron clearance but by obtaining blood samples over a period of 2 weeks, the percent of the original dose absorbed by the red cells can be determined. This percentage is high and rapid in active marrow turnovers. It is low and slow in myelofibrosis and aplastic anemia.

■ **Describe the radioactive fat studies.**

A complete fat (triolein) labeled with radioactive iodine is given orally. If there is a fat-splitting pancreatic enzyme (lipase) present, and if there is intestinal integrity, much of this fat will be absorbed. This level of absorption can be tested by collecting stool and determining the low level of residual radioactivity or by collecting blood and determining the elevated level of radioactivity over a period of 4 to 6 hours. If either lipase or intestinal integrity is impaired, the blood levels are low and the stool levels will be high. To distinguish between the two possible deficiencies, the test is repeated using a fatty acid (oleic acid) labeled with radioactive iodine. This fatty acid does not require lipase for absorption. If the blood level remains low or the stool level high, poor intestinal integrity or malabsorption is indicated. If the blood level is high and the stool is low in radioactivity, the indication is poor pancreatic function.

CHAPTER 6

Microbiology and immunology

SILAS G. FARMER

■ **What are the different sterilization methods commonly used in the laboratory? Name one application for each.**

Autoclaving, or moist heat under pressure (15 lbs, 15 minutes), is the best method of sterilization of materials that are not adversely affected by this treatment. Ethylene oxide sterilization is the method of choice for plastics and other solids that cannot withstand high heat. Filtration through membrane filters or fritted glass filters are to be used for sterilizing liquids such as carbohydrate solutions, serum, and urea solutions.

■ **What is meant by selective, differential, and enrichment media?**

A selective medium is one in which some agent has been added to offer a selective advantage to one or more organisms. Hence Thayer-Martin medium with VCN offers a selective advantage to *Neisseria gonorrhoeae* and *N. meningitidis* because the antibiotics V (vancomycin), C (colistin), and N (nystatin) effectively inhibit most other *Neisseria* species as well as many other bacteria and yeast which may be found in reproductive cultures.

A differential medium permits the differentiation between two organisms with respect to one or more characteristics. For example, a simple carbohydrate such as glucose and an indicator which changes color upon lowering the pH following growth permits the differentiation between those that can and those that cannot ferment (or oxidize) that carbohydrate.

An enrichment medium contains ingredients to enrich the formulation, usually to permit the isolation of the more fastidious microorganisms. Enrichments may be vitamins, yeast extract, serum, or other growth-stimulating components.

Media used in the clinical laboratory frequently contain one or more of the above characteristics. Hence the Thayer-Martin is both a selective medium because of the VCN and an enrichment medium because of the Iso-Vitalex additive.

■ **What is coagulase?**

Coagulase is a kinase produced by most pathogenic *Staphylococcus aureus* which, if allowed to interact with a plasma factor (coagulase reacting factor or CRF), will produce a thrombokinase-like active principle, which will convert fibrinogen into fibrin and result in clotting. However, unlike thrombokinase, the CRF does not require calcium for its formation. The extracellular coagulase, or "free coagulase," is best detected with rabbit plasma in a test tube.

The "bound coagulase" or clumping factor does not require CRF, is performed as a slide test, and may be detected with human plasma.

Although good correlation is observed between the two methods, a negative slide test is best followed up with the tube test.

■ **What is ONPG, and why is it used?**

ONPG is o-nitrophenyl-β-D-galactopyranoside and is the reagent used to detect the enzyme β-galactosidase.

Lactose fermentation requires the presence of β-galactosidase, an intracellular enzyme, and a permease. In the absence of permease, potentially lactose-fermenting organisms are unable to do so because of the inability of the lactose to enter the cell. In the ONPG test, the organisms are grown on a lactose-containing medium that encourages the development of β-galactoside permease mutants. Thus the presence of potential lactose fermenters which otherwise might be considered as late fermenters or even nonfermenters may be detected. In the positive test, β-galactosidase splits o-nitrophenol, a yellow compound, from ONPG.

Although not recommended as a substitute for the lactose fermentation test, it is nevertheless useful detecting late lactose fermenting *E. coli, Klebsiella,* and other members of *Enterobacteriaceae.* Another useful application is in differentiating *Salmonella* (ONPG negative) from *Citrobacter* and *Arizona* (both ONPG positive).

■ **What enzyme is produced by an indole positive organism and how is it detected?**

Tryptophanase is detected by means of the widely used procedure known as Kovac's method. The reagent is prepared by dissolving p-dimethylaminobenzaldehyde in amyl or isoamyl alcohol, which is then acidified with concentrated HCl. When this reagent is added to a culture containing indole, a deep red color develops.

■ **What portion of the pneumococcus is associated with virulence?**

In the mouse model, the presence of the capsule has been shown to be the virulence factor. A few encapsulated pneumococci will produce a fatal disease, whereas as many as 1×10^6 nonencapsulated ones (derived from the same serotype) will not.

In man, phagocytosis is retarded by the presence of a capsule. However, the virulence factors are poorly understood but one is thought to be a neuraminidase.

■ **What differences exist between alpha and beta hemolysis other than the color surrounding the colony?**

Beta hemolysis is characterized by complete hemolysis of red blood cells surrounding the colony. The two hemolysins are oxygen-labile streptolysin O and the oxygen-stable streptolysin S. Although only streptolysin S produces hemolysis around surface colonies, both O and S produce hemolysis in the deep cut section of the blood agar or in the test tube suspension of red blood cells.

The alpha-hemolytic streptococci are surrounded by a narrow zone of incomplete hemolysis in which unhemolyzed red blood cells adjacent to the colony may be seen microscopically. This zone may be surrounded by a zone of complete hemolysis. Green discoloration of the medium surrounding the colony, because of the formation of an unidentified reductant of hemoglobin, may occur with some species of red blood cells under certain conditions of incubation.

■ **Explain the meaning and processing of a blood agar plate with beta hemolysis only in the cut portion.**

The most probable explanation is that the organism is a beta-hemolytic streptococcus that is producing only streptolysin O and not streptolysin S. The specimen should be handled in the same manner as any other beta-hemolytic streptococcus.

■ **Why is it clinically useful to group beta-hemolytic streptococci?**

Beta-hemolytic streptococci represent a very heterogeneous group with diverse clinical significance. The most important is group A in causing human disease. Recently, group B has been increasingly associated with neonatal infection. Some members of group D comprise the enterococci. The clinical significance of other groups varies greatly. Although group A streptococci are exquisitely sensitive to penicillin, some other streptococci are quite different in their antibiotic susceptibility.

■ **Which serotypes of group A streptococcus pyogenes are associated with acute glomerulonephritis?**

M protein types 4, 12, 25, and 49 have the greatest association, although occasionally a new M type has been described.

■ **Which streptococci are of increasing concern in neonatal infection?**

Streptococcus agalactae, or group B of the Lancefield classification, is significant in neonatal infection.

■ **What are enterococci, and why is it clinically important to identify these organisms?**

Enterococci are enteric streptococci belonging to the Lancefield group D. *S. fecalis, S. fecalis* var. *liquefaciens,* and *S. fecium* are nonhemolytic, but *S. fecalis* var. *zymogenes* and *S. durans* produce beta hemolysis on blood agar. Some members of the serologic group D are not enterococci, i.e., *S. bovis* and *S. equinas.*

The enterococci are not as sensitive to penicillin as are the group A streptococci. The antibiotic dosage must be adjusted upward to effectively treat infections caused by the enterococci, i.e., endocarditis.

■ **What test can be used in the laboratory to differentiate between streptococci and staphylococci?**

Catalase is the test of choice. The staphylococci and micrococci produce catalase, which is easily detected by adding a drop of 3% hydrogen peroxide to the bacteria and observing bubble formation. Inasmuch as blood contains small amounts of catalase, care must be exercised when testing organisms growing on blood agar.

■ **Differentiate among *Edwardsiella tarda, Arizona hinshawii, Citrobacter fruendii,* and most *Salmonella* organisms.**

Citrobacter differs from the rest of these organisms in that it lacks lysine decarboxylase. Of the remaining, *E. tarda* differs from the arizona and salmonella by being indole positive. A positive malonate differentiates the arizona from the salmonella. Of course, the latter two could be differentiated on a serologic basis.

■ **Are members of the family Enterobacteriaceae only enteric pathogens?**

No. Some members are plant pathogens, and some produce infection only when found outside of the gut. The most significant enteric pathogens are Salmonella, Shigella, enteropathogenic *E. coli*, and *Yersinia enterocolytica*. The recent inclusion of Yersinia into the family brings along *Y. pestis (Pasteurella pestis)* and adds a whole new dimension to the clinical syndromes associated with this family.

■ **The biochemical reaction on an enteric organism is as follows: negative reactions for phenylalanine deaminase, H_2S, gas from glucose, lysine decarboxylase, lactose fermentation, citrate utilization, and malonate. It is positive for ornithine decarboxylase and urease, and is motile at 20° C. What might the organism be and of what clinical significance is this organism?**

An aerogenic, lactose-negative, urease-producing gram-negative bacillus which is motile only at 25° C is very suggestive of *Yersinia enterocolitica*. Yersinia produce mainly enteric syndromes such as cervical adenitis, enteritis, enterocolitis, terminal ileitis, appendicitis, and diarrhea. Occasionally cases of septicemia and even less often cases of meningitis have been observed.

■ **What is the clinical importance of *Pseudomonas aeruginosa?***

Members of the genus *Pseudomonas* are widespread in nature and usually cause little concern for the healthy individual. In the burn patient, *P. aeruginosa* rapidly colonizes the eschar because of antibiotic therapy used to suppress the staphylococci, and frequently leads to fatal infection. Nosocomial infections, especially pulmonary disease in patients on respiration equipment for extended periods of time and renal disease in patients who have had instrumentation, continue to cause concern to infectious disease control committees in hospitals.

■ **Which anaerobe produces a black pigment and what is the clinical significance of this organism?**

Bacteroides melaninogenicus produces a black pigment. It has been associated with infections of the female genital tract, bone and joint infections, liver and pulmonary abscesses, intestinal lesions, and infections of the mouth and gums.

■ **What differences are noted between *Mycobacterium tuberculosis* and *M. kansasii?***

M. tuberculosis usually appears as a dry colorless to buff colony on inspissated egg media and is characterized by producing niacin and reducing nitrates to nitrites.

Although *M. kansasii* is usually buff-colored when first seen, it is photochromogenic, producing a yellow color following exposure to light and continued incubation. The colony is usually smooth and is characterized by no niacin production but by reduction of nitrates. It must be recalled that some strains of *M. tuberculosis* that are resistant to INH may be unable to produce niacin.

■ **Is *Mycobacterium tuberculosis* resistant to heat?**

Although *M. tuberculosis* may remain viable in culture media and dried sputum for up to eight months and is quite resistant to chemical disinfection, it is as sensitive to moist heat as are other vegetative forms of bacteria. Therefore pasteurization temperatures are effective in eliminating the tubercle bacillus from milk and milk products.

■ **What are L-forms and how may they be cultivated?**

L-forms are cell wall deficient forms of bacteria that may be induced by antibiotics which act upon cell wall synthesis (such as penicillin) and complement, for example. They are osmotically fragile and can only survive and reproduce in a hypertonic environment.

Nutritional media adequate to support the parental type of the species and containing 0.3 M sucrose or 20% serum will usually grow most L-forms.

■ **What is the clinical significance of cell wall deficient (CWD) or L-forms?**

Although CWD or L-forms are not capable of producing disease, they may revert back to the parental type upon removal from the environment which induced them (i.e., discontinuing the antibiotic therapy), with the resulting virulence and pathogenicity of the parental type.

■ **How can *Mycoplasma pneumoniae* be isolated?**

Mycoplasma organisms are really bacteria without cell walls and therefore must be cultivated in a hypertonic medium. The use of PPLO medium base, enriched with 20% serum, yeast extract, and agents to restrict the growth of other oral and pharyngeal organisms, i.e., penicillin, amphotericin B, and thallium acetate, will usually suffice. An anaerobic atmosphere with added 5% carbon dioxide is preferable. Inasmuch as 7 to 9 days may be required for isolation, plates must be taped to prevent desiccation during the incubation.

■ **In what ways can disease-producing microorganisms be transmitted?**

Fracastorius de Verona in 1535 said that the seeds of disease could be transmitted (1) by direct contact, (2) by fomites, and (3) ad distans or at great distances via aerosol. He was right! We have added new vehicles such as frozen foods, transfused blood, and venipuncture needles, but we have not added to the basic understanding of disease transmission.

■ **What organisms may cause food poisoning?**

Food poisoning may be caused by *Clostridium botulinum* and *Staphylococcus aureus*. In food poisoning the viable organism need not be present to produce the toxicosis.

■ **What is food infection?**

Food infection is a gastrointestinal disease caused by the ingestion of rather large numbers of viable bacteria in food. This type of disorder may be found with *Salmonella, Clostridium perfringens,* and *Vibrio parahemolyticus.* In contrast, food poisoning caused by *C. botulinum* or *S. aureus* does not require the ingestion of viable bacteria but rather just their toxins and is a primary toxicosis.

■ **What is the difference between bacteremia and septicemia?**

Bacteremia merely designates the presence of bacteria in the bloodstream. This may be a simple transient bacteremia following a vigorous tooth brushing or a significant one leading to symptomatology of sepsis. Septicemia implies disease and therefore symptomatology, i.e., fever, toxic reactions with or without shock, and so on.

■ **What guidelines are reasonable to follow in the collection of blood cultures with respect to the number, timing, and so on?**

Blood cultures are indicated in the febrile patient during the actual fever. Most organisms may be recovered from the bloodstream at any time during the bacteremia. However, some, such as *Brucella,* tend to be tissue parasites and are shed periodically. For this reason several blood cultures should be drawn.

The most reasonable guidelines suggest a routine of three blood cultures drawn over the period of 1 working day. More frequent blood cultures, over a longer period of time, may be required if brucellosis is suspected.

■ **What is Liquoid or SPS and what effects does it exert in the blood culture?**

Liquoid or SPS is sodium polyanethol sulfonate. It is an anticoagulant of much less toxicity than oxalate or citrate; when incorporated into blood culture broth at a final concentration of 0.05% it is anticomplementary and inhibits both the bactericidal action of blood and the phagocytic activity of leukocytes. Bacteria survive more readily in Liquoid than in citrated blood and are more readily recovered in broth cultures.

■ **What visible signs are suggestive of bacterial growth in a blood culture bottle? How would you handle a bottle that did not display these signs?**

Turbidity in the supernate, white colonies lying on top of the sedimented cells, and early hemolysis are all suggestive of bacterial growth. However, *Brucella, Neisseria meningitidis, Haemophilus influenzae,* yeast, and others may not produce sufficient growth (greater than 1×10^6 organisms/ml) to produce turbidity.

Bottles that do not show the above characteristics should be subcultured to enriched agar at 24 or 48 hours and again before discarding as "no growth" to detect these positives that are not grossly apparent.

■ **What bacteria may be isolated from blood cultures?**

Almost any bacterium may be isolated from blood cultures. Some of the isolates may be virulent pathogens such as *Staphylococcus aureus, Escherichia coli, Proteus,* or others capable of producing sepsis in any individual. Others may be low-grade pathogens that usually infect only the compromised host, such as *Staphylococcus epidermidis, Flavobacterium,* or *Citrobacter fruendii.* Some isolates may represent only the indigenous flora of the skin and not a bacteremia. This may result from inadequate preparation of the skin prior to collection of the specimen.

■ **What explanation might be offered for the frequent isolation of low-grade pathogens, or opportunists, from blood culture bottles?**

Organisms that comprise the indigenous flora of the skin (i.e., *Staphylococcus epidermidis* and diphtheroids) are frequently recovered from the blood culture bottle because the venipuncture site was not properly disinfected.

■ **A patient is suspected of having typhoid fever. What specimens taken at what times are indicated for laboratory analysis?**

During the first week, most patients have septicemia and a positive blood culture may be obtained. About 25% of these patients will also have a positive urine culture during this time. Positive stool cultures may be obtained about the second week of illness, and about that time agglutinins appear in the serum. A second agglutination titer should be obtained, about 10 days to 2 weeks after the first, in order to demonstrate a fourfold or greater increase in titer.

Of course, not all of these procedures may be required. A positive blood culture would suffice. However, if the blood culture is negative or if the patient had passed that phase of illness in which septicemia is a component, the other procedure would be indicated.

■ **Anaerobic bacteria may cause serious pulmonary infection. Which specimens are acceptable and which are not acceptable for anaerobic culture?**

A transtracheal aspirate is the only specimen that can produce meaningful clinical results as of this date. Potentially, the bronchial brush technique may offer good specimens. Sputum or bronchial washings are invariably contaminated with the indigenus anaerobic oral flora and are not acceptable for anaerobic culture.

■ **What are the best methods for digestion and processing sputum cultures for *Mycobacterium tuberculosis?***

Sodium hydroxide and trisodium phosphate were used for many years to digest the mucus and decontaminate the specimen. However, the best method is the use of NAC (n-acetyl cystine) and sodium hydroxide.

■ **Discuss how you would handle a cloudy spinal fluid in the microbiology laboratory.**

Any spinal fluid with an abnormal white blood count should be processed promptly. A gram stained smear should be made of the sediment and if bacteria are seen the report should be called immediately to the physician. If bacteria are present, the choice of media is more apparent. However, if cultures are to be set up without this knowledge, inoculate media that would support the growth of *N. meningitis,* pneumococcus, *H. influenzae,* and streptococci. A blood agar and chocolate agar with enrichment incubated at 35 to 37° C in 5 to 10% CO_2 should suffice.

Cultures for fungi or *M. tuberculosis* are usually not performed unless specifically requested.

■ **Which is the better atmosphere for incubating blood agar plates from respiratory cultures, O_2 or CO_2?**

Carbon dioxide is preferable for several reasons. Some pneumococcal strains are capnophilic (require CO_2) and would be missed if not grown in that atmosphere.

■ **What organisms are most frequently associated with primary urinary tract infection in the female?**

Usually *E. coli* (85%), because of the shortness of the female urethra and the anatomic proximity to the fecal flora.

■ **A gram stained smear of exudate from a cervicofacial draining nodule reveals gram positive branching filaments. What clinical diagnosis is suggested?**

A clinical diagnosis of actinomycosis is suggested. *Actinomyces israelii* and *A. naeslundii* are the two most frequently encountered species.

■ **Trench mouth or Vincent's angina is a fusospirochetal symbiotic disease. How would you process a request and what would you look for? What is the limitation of the procedure?**

A smear from the diseased portion stained with Wright's, carbol fuchsin, or some other strong stain and examined for fusiform bacilli and *Borellia* is the proper procedure. Inasmuch as the organisms that cause Vincent's angina are indigenous oral flora, they are of significance only when they are present in large numbers.

An alternative method of examination would be to make a hanging drop examination from the affected area and view with darkfield. *Treponema microdentium* would also be seen by this method.

The diagnosis of Vincent's angina is a clinical one and cannot be made by the laboratory solely on the examination of the smears.

■ **What are some frequent causes of bacterial pneumonia in the adult?**

Streptococcus (Diplococcus) pneumoniae continues to be the most frequently encountered species, occurring in about 75% of the patients. About 10% are caused by various gram negative bacilli of the family Enterobacteriaceae (i.e., *Klebsiella pneumoniae, E. coli, Enterobacter*) and about 7% are staphylococcal in origin. The other may be *Haemophilus influenzae, Mycoplasma pneumoniae,* or anaerobic gram negative bacilli.

■ **What is the significance of many epithelial cells in a smear from a specimen labelled "sputum?"**

The presence of many epithelial cells indicates that the specimen was contaminated with saliva and is therefore an improper specimen for processing. The bacteria encountered represent the indigenous oral flora rather than the organisms involved in the patient's respiratory tract infection. The simple expedient of rinsing the mouth prior to sputum collection will do much to remove the saliva contamination. However, the transtracheal aspiration is bacteriologically the best for processing.

■ **Describe proper collection and examination technique for the flagellated protozoon that causes a venereal disease.**

Trichomonas vaginalis is the only trichomonad found in the vagina or urethral tract. Diagnosis may be made by preparing saline wet mounts of vaginal exudate and examining with the microscope. The typical nervous, jerky, trichomonal movement and the characteristic undulating membrane readily identify this protozoon. Some authors have reported better luck with culture techniques, however.

■ **Describe a positive smear for gonorrhea in a male with acute urethritis.**

The uncomplicated gonorrhea in the male is characterized by acute urethritis with a marked purulent reaction. A gram stained smear would reveal many PMN's with many intracellular and extracellular gram negative diplococci. Although this is the typical picture, the organism *Neisseria gonorrhoeae* cannot be legally identified by smear alone. The report of the smear should contain the observation, but should contain the phrase . . . "which is morphologically similar to *N. gonorrhoeae*."

■ **Why is it not a good idea to diagnose gonorrhea from a cervical or vaginal smear?**

Many bacteria may be seen on smears from these areas and some of the gram-negative bacilli may resemble *N. gonorrhoeae* morphologically. In addition, many women are asymptomatic and *N. gonorrhoeae* are present in low numbers. Culture of multiple sites such as cervical, anal, vaginal, and pharyngeal areas are necessary to detect all cases of gonorrhea.

■ **What bacteria would you normally expect to find in the vagina?**

Women of childbearing age might have *Lactobacillus, Corynebacterium, Staphylococcus, Micrococcus,* streptococci (beta-hemolytic *S. fecalis,* other aerobic streptococci, and *Peptostreptococcus*), *E. coli, Proteus, Candida,* and *C. perfringens.*

■ **A patient is seen with a shallow ulcer on his penis and swollen lymph nodes or buboes. What infections might this suggest?**

This might be lymphogranuloma venereum, granuloma inguinale, or chancroid.

■ **What precautions should be followed in preparing slide mounts of fungi that have a white aerial mycelium?**

Many laboratory contaminants, dermatophytes, and systemic fungi are characterized by white aerial mycelium. Inasmuch as the identity of the fungus cannot be ascertained with accuracy by the gross appearance of the mycelium, it is best to handle all specimens as if they were highly infectious. The use of laminar flow hoods and the practice of "wetting-down" the aerial mycelium by carefully overlaying the slant with sterile water or saline should be practiced. The distribution of aerial spores is to be avoided. Although the distribution of contaminant spores creates only laboratory contamination, the spores of *Coccidioides immitis, Blastomyces dermatitidis,* and *Histoplasma capsulatum* are highly infectious to laboratory personnel.

■ **What methods may be used to quantitate gentamicin?**

The classic tube dilution method is not adequate for the assay of gentamicin because it requires too much time (18 to 24 hours) and it is not sensitive enough (serial twofold decrements) for the clinical evaluation of patients.

A rapid (3- to 4-hour) procedure by Sabath, which measures the ability of gentamicin (or any other aminoglycoside) to inhibit the germination of *Bacillus subtilis* spores, is reproducible within $\pm 10\%$ and results are available before the next scheduled dose of antibiotic. This procedure is easily performed even in the small clinical laboratory and the plates used in the assay may be stored in the refrigerator for several weeks. The most recent method available for the assay of gentamicin, and one that overcomes the problem inherent in the situation in which the patient is on several antibiotics, is a sensitive, specific, and rapid method which requires minute amounts of serum. An R-factor-mediated enzyme that adenylates gentamicin has been employed in a radioactive assay. ATP serves as the source of the adenyl group transferred to the antibiotic during the reaction. Adenylated gentamicin, but not ATP, is positively charged and therefore binds to the negatively charged phosphocellulose (PC) paper. When aliquots of the mixture, containing ^{14}C-ATP, are pipetted onto PC paper and washed to eliminate nonspecifically bound radioactivity, the PC bound radioactivity measures adenylated antibiotic.

■ **What is the clinical usefulness of a serum gentamicin assay?**

Gentamicin is relatively toxic. It causes ototoxicity in approximately 2.3% of patients but renal damage in fewer patients. The ototoxicity is usually correlated with previous otologic status, prior therapy with other ototoxic drugs, age, and the serum concentrations. However, since gentamicin is excreted primarily by the kidneys, serum concentrations reflect the dosage, route of administration, interval between doses, and renal function of the patient.

Most dosage schedules aim to attain a concentration of about 4 μg/ml gentamicin in serum. However, concentrations above 10 to 12 μg/ml are considered potentially toxic.

Although serum concentration correlates with renal function, the half-life cannot be calculated from creatinine clearance or serum creatinine concentrations in the acutely ill or dehydrated individual or one who has minimal muscle mass. Thus a rapid and accurate serum assay is needed to avoid toxic levels of gentamicin.

■ **What do the terms MIC and MBC designate and of what clinical use are they?**

They represent minimum inhibitory concentration (MIC) and minimum bactericidal concentration (MBC), respectively. They are usually used to designate the concentration of antibiotic that is required to inhibit or kill an organism. This information is useful in initiating or quantitating antibiotic therapy, especally if the treatment is to be given over a protracted period.

■ **Discuss the principle, procedure, and value of the Schlicter test.**

The Schlicter test is a twofold tube dilution test to determine the total killing power of the serum against the organism causing the patient's infection. This test measures the effects of one or more antibiotics, complement, or other cidal agents in the patient's serum. A cidal effect at a serum dilution of fourfold is acceptable, but an eightfold cidal titer is preferable.

Those tubes in which no visible growth is observed should be subcultured to antibiotic-free media to ascertain whether the organisms have been killed or were only inhibited. The results can be expressed as the bacteriostatic titer (highest serum dilution that inhibits growth) and the bactericidal titer (highest serum dilution that kills the organism).

■ **Which organisms cannot be tested for antibiotic susceptibility by the Kirby-Bauer disc diffusion method?**

The Kirby-Bauer test was devised for the rapidly growing aerobic bacteria. This procedure cannot be used for slow-growing bacteria such as *M. tuberculosis* or any of the anaerobic bacteria. Atmospheres such as carbon dioxide change the pH of the medium to acid and affect the action of some antibiotics.

■ **What variables might influence the zone size in the Kirby-Bauer antibiotic sensitivity test?**

Possible sources of variability include the age and size of the inoculum, the manner in which the plate is inoculated, the antibiotic content of the disc, medium concentration, pH, moisture content of agar, thickness of agar, length of incubation, and method of illuminating and reading zones.

■ **What is the usefulness of the Maloney test?**

The Maloney test is used to detect hypersensitivity to the diphtheria toxoid. It is used in the adult to prevent anaphylactic shock upon administration of the toxoid.

■ **What is the Schick test?**

The Schick test is an intradermal skin test used to detect the presence of circulating antibodies to the diphtheria toxin. Although not correlated 100% with immunity, for practical purposes it is usually assumed that if no redness and induration appear after the injection of 0.1 ml containing 1/50 MLD, the individual has 1/500 to 1/250 units of antitoxin/ml and thus is able to protect against infection by the diphtheria bacillus.

■ **What is the Neufeld-Quellung reaction and with which organisms may it be applied?**

The Neufeld-Quellung reaction is a swelling of the polysaccharide capsular material in the presence of homologous antibody. Any organism with a capsular polysaccharide may demonstrate this reaction. *Streptococcus (Diplococcus) pneumoniae, Klebsiella,* and *Haemophilus* are frequently typed by this procedure.

■ **What is the purpose of heating the bacterial suspension when performing some agglutination reactions with the salmonelleae?**

Some salmonella contain a Vi antigen, which is an envelope antigen that, if present in sufficient amount, can mask the detection of the underlying somatic or O antigens. These envelope antigens are thermolabile and thus destroyed by heat to reveal the O antigens. It is a good practice to test the bacterial suspension with anti-Vi antiserum.

■ **What is the value of quality control in microbiology?**

Quality control means that all the factors which are important for the accurate analysis are known to be performing properly. The specimen has been properly collected, correctly processed, and plated on media that will support characteristic growth in a known environment. The personnel can recognize the growth and identify the significant isolate with media and reagents which are known to give accurate results. The report is transmitted to proper recording areas without error. In general, you are confident that the analysis has been correct and complete.

■ **Many laboratories use TSI, KIA, or RDS for enteric bacteriology. What is the meaning of "acid/acid," "alk/acid," and so on on these media?**

These media are characterized by the incorporation of two or three carbohydrates in different concentrations in an agar slant containing an indicator. Usually glucose is present in 0.1% concentration and lactose or lactose and sucrose in 1.0% concentrations.

The slant represents aerobic growth conditions, whereas the butt is more anaerobic. If only the CHO present in low concentration, i.e., glucose (in the above examples) was fermented, the entire tube would become acid (yellow with a phenol red indicator) initially, but in the aerobic slant the reaction would proceed to completion through the Krebs cycle to form CO_2 and water. At this time (24 hours) the slant would appear as if it had not changed (it would appear red or alkaline). The butt, lacking oxygen, could not pass beyond lactic acid or pyruvic acid and the butt portion would be acid (yellow) because of the accumulation of the intermediary organic acids resulting from the degradation or fermentation of the CHO.

However, if the CHO present in greater concentration, 1.0% (lactose and/or sucrose), was fermented, the reaction in the slant portion could not proceed to completion for several days and therefore would appear yellow, as would the butt.

■ **How could you isolate and identify pathogenic *Neisseria* from the upper respiratory tract?**

The two most important *Neisseria* in the URT are *Neisseria meningitidis* and *N. gonorrhoeae*. *N. gonorrhoeae* may produce gonococcal pharyngitis and *N. meningitidis* may produce local inflammation of the pharynx prior to any central nervous system involvement or bacteremia. Both organisms will grow readily on Thayer-Martin medium with Iso-Vitalex enrichment and containing VCN in an atmosphere of 5 to 10% carbon dioxide at 35 to 37° C.

■ **What is the significance of a colony count on urine and how may this count be determined?**

It has been determined that rather low counts (organisms/ml) may be found under normal conditions and represent contamination of the urethra with indigenous flora. However, counts of 10^5 and greater are usually significant, indicating either current infection or a propensity to infectious sequelae, such as pyelonephritis, if the patient is asymptomatic.

■ **How would you culture a stool specimen from a patient with suspected bacterial diarrhea if there were no history of consumption of raw clams or travel to "cholera countries?"**

Promptness in processing is indicated. Make a suspension of the stool specimen in sterile saline and inoculate agar plates of MacConkey's, brilliant green, XLD, salmonella-shigella, Hektoen, or other appropriate formulations. Inoculate gram negative broth with part of the stool specimen for enrichment and subculture to appropriate media after overnight incubation.

Colonies resembling *Salmonella, Shigella,* and enteropathogenic *E. coli* (if from a child) should be picked and inoculated onto differential media for biochemical identification and serologic typing, if indicated.

■ **Name several commonly encountered bacteria from spinal fluid and the age groups associated with each.**

Neisseria meningitidis causes a rather severe meningitis, worldwide in distribution, which occurs in both sporadic and epidemic forms. Although all ages may be involved, cases are more frequently seen among infants and young children. The disease is endemic in large cities and epidemic periods may be seen in this country which coincide with major population movement and recruit training camps. In one reported series of 258 cases over a 3-year period, 48% occurred between 0 and 4 years, 17% between 5 and 14, 14% between 15 and 29, and the remaining 23% from the age of 30 or more.

Haemophilus influenzae is the most common form of suppurative meningitis between the neonatal period and age 6, the period when *N. meningitidis* is not epidemic. *H. influenzae* is the most common cause of bacterial meningitis. About 40% of the cases of *H. influenzae* meningitis occur before age 1 and another 53% between 1 and 4 years of age. The remaining 7% are scattered over the remaining years.

Pneumococcal meningitis is the third most common variety of acute bacterial meningitis. It is seen more commonly among infants and the elderly.

If one looks at neonatal meningitis, one sees a variety of bacterial etiologies. In one study of 94 cases in Los Angeles, during a 6-year period no bacteria were isolated and identified in 22 of the cases. Of the identified species, in decreasing order of occurrence were *E. coli,* unidentified gram negative bacilli of the family Enterobacteriaceae designated *Paracolon* (12), *Klebsiella* or *Enterobacter* (10), *Streptococcus* (8), *Proteus* (5), *Listeria monocytogenes* (5), *Salmonella* (3), *Staphylococcus epidermidis* (3), *Diplococcus pneumoniae* (2), *Haemophilus influenzae* (2), and *Pseudomonas* and *Mimae,* 1 each. Thus in this study of meningitis in the neonate, of the bacteria isolated, over 70% of the cases belong to the family Enterobacteriaceae.

■ **What is meant by "redox" potential and of what use is it in the laboratory?**

Redox potential is a term used to express the oxidation-reduction potential or Eh (expressed as positive or negative millivolts) of the environment. The milieu of man varies greatly with respect to its Eh. Thus normal tissue has an Eh of about +120 mV while the Eh of pus is about −230 mV. For reference, the Eh of hydrogen is −420 mV.

Organisms vary greatly in their aerotolerance; thus aerobes such as *Pseudomonas* will not grow in a medium with a very low Eh. At the other end of the spectrum, strict anaerobes such as *Clostridium tetani* will not grow and sporulate if the Eh is too high. Most organisms, while they are considered aerobes, will also grow at very low Eh values and thus are termed facultative.

When one desires to isolate strict anaerobes from an abscess, one should select the conditions that give a very low Eh value, such as prereduced anaerobically sterilized (PRAS) medium with an Eh of about −150 mV. The pH of the medium will greatly influence the Eh value. The Eh value will become 60 mV more negative for each unit increase in the pH. Thus, a medium with an Eh value of $+100$ mV at pH 6 would have Eh values of $+40$ and -20 mV at pH values of 7 and 8, respectively.

■ **How does the Gas-Pak hydrogen-CO_2 generator work?**

Gas-Pak (BBL) is a commercially available envelope containing a hydrogen-producing sodium borohydride tablet and a citric acid + sodium bicarbonate tablet which produces carbon dioxide. It is activated by adding 10 ml of water. A catalyst, active at room temperature, consists of alumina pellets coated with 0.5% palladium. Free molecular oxygen is thus combined with the hydrogen to form water and reduce the redox potential of the atmosphere sufficiently to support those organisms termed "anaerobes."

■ **What genera comprise the family Enterobacteriaceae?**

Escherichia, Edwardsiella, Salmonella, Arizona, Shigella, Citrobacter, Klebsiella, Enterobacter, Serratia, Proteus, Providencia, Yersinia, and *Pectobacterium* comprise the Enterobacteriaceae.

■ **What is the laboratory importance of bacterial dissociation?**

Most bacterial dissociation is of the S-R type (smooth to rough), with the resulting loss of superficial "O" antigens. When these are necessary for antigenic analysis, i.e., typhoid bacillus or other Enterobacteriaceae agglutination, fluorescent antibody identification of *Bordetella pertussis,* or capsular typing of pneumococci, it is impossible to demonstrate the expected antigen-antibody reaction. Inasmuch as the S-R dissociation is usually not complete, it may be reversed by animal passage. For example, when a mixture of S and R forms are injected into an animal, the R (rough) forms are rapidly phagocytized and the S (smooth, virulent) forms persist and can be isolated.

■ **What effect does contaminating saliva have upon the microbial content of sputum?**

Many organisms are found as indigenous oral flora and can be recovered from saliva. Many of these may represent only the transient flora. However, it is difficult to impossible to assign a role to many of the organisms solely upon identification. Thus a *Klebsiella pneumoniae* from saliva has the same characteristics as a *Klebsiella pneumoniae* from lobar pneumonia. Of significance also is the fact that some enzymes in saliva will mask the detection of or lyse some bacteria such as *Streptococcus (Diplococcus) pneumoniae.*

■ **What effect does storage at room temperature for 4 or more hours have upon the microbial content of sputum?**

The concentration of contaminating or nonpathogenic *Staphylococcus epidermidis*, *Neisseria* sp., *Streptococcus viridans*, and potentially pathogenic *Streptococcus pneumoniae*, *Haemophilus influenzae*, *Klebsiella*, *Enterobacter*, and *E. coli* increases 1 to 3 logs/ml upon storage at room temperature for 4 or more hours. The concentration of some potential pathogens changes from a clinically insignificant 1×10^3 to a significant 1×10^6 or more organisms/ml.

■ **What test is useful to differentiate the *Proteus* and *Providencia* from other members of the family Enterobacteriaceae and from each other?**

Both *Proteus* and *Providencia* elaborate the enzyme phenylalanine deaminase and thus are separated from most of the other members of this family. They may be differentiated from one another with the urease test; the *Providencia* lack this enzyme.

Although some strains of *Enterobacter agglomerans* may produce a phenylalanine deaminase, they may be differentiated from these two genera by fermenting arabinose and being yellow (75%).

■ **How do endotoxins differ from exotoxins?**

Most exotoxins are readily released into the substrate, are quite specific in their action, are very antigenic, are readily neutralized by their homologous antibody, and are thermolabile.

A notable exception is the thermostable enterotoxin of *Staphylococcus aureus*, the exotoxin that causes staphylococcal food poisoning. Toxins, which are termed endotoxins, are very similar to each other in their action regardless of bacterial origin. They are weakly antigenic, not readily released from the bacterial cell, relatively heat stable, and produced primarily by gram negative bacilli. Endotoxins are less toxic than exotoxins but if administered in sufficient quantity can cause fever and irreversible shock and can exert an effect upon nonspecific immunity.

■ **In what manner are the enterotoxins of *Staphylococcus aureus* different from other exotoxins?**

There are three emetic toxins produced by certain strains of *S. aureus* which are thermostable. They will survive heating to 100° C for 30 minutes. Another way to visualize this resistance to heat is to consider a chocolate eclair filled with custard and staphylococci with one of the enterotoxins after boiling for half an hour. You can imagine the appearance of the eclair—but the enterotoxins will still be present and active.

■ **What organisms may cause "gas" production with necrosis of tissue?**

The gas gangrene group of *Clostridia* such as *C. perfringens, C. septicum, C. novyi, C. histolyticum,* and *C. bifermentans.* In addition, members of the Enterobacteriaceae such as *E. coli* may also be included. A gassy necrotic cellulitis caused by anaerobes or symbiotic action of *Peptostreptococcus* and *Staphylococcus aureus* may also be encountered.

■ **What two species of *Corynebacterium* elaborate a diphtheria toxin and how may they be differentiated?**

Corynebacterium diphtheriae, var. *mitis, gravis,* and *intermedius* and *C. ulcerans* elaborate a diphtheria toxin. Pleomorphism is more pronounced in *C. ulcerans;* it does not reduce nitrate to nitrites, but hydrolyzes urea and slowly liquefies gelatin.

■ **What is lockjaw and how can it be prevented?**

Lockjaw is one of the clinical manifestations of tetanus, which is an intoxication with the exotoxin of *Clostridium tetani.* It is characterized by intense, severe muscle spasms. The toxin, known as tetanospasmin, is among the most potent bacterial toxins known. Spores of *C. tetani* are introduced by contamination of a wound. The transformation of spores into toxin-producing vegetative forms requires a lower redox (oxidation-reduction) potential than is present in normal tissues. Necrosis resulting from the trauma or the presence of other bacteria can lower the redox potential sufficiently. The organism has little or no invasive capacity but the toxin is absorbed into the CNS, bloodstream, and muscles. The major clinical manifestation of tetanus is muscular rigidity; when this involves the facial or masseter muscles, it is referred to as lockjaw or trismus. However, the toxicity will usually progress to general tetanus and cause violent contractions of the neck, trunk, and limb muscles.

Clinical tetanus is preventable by immunization with tetanus toxoid.

■ **Differentiate among the genera *Listeria, Erysipelothrix,* and *Corynebacterium.***

The organisms of all three of these genera are gram positive bacilli and to the average person could not be differentiated on a morphologic basis.

E. rhusiopathiae can *be* separated from the catalase negative *C. pyogenes* and *C. haemolyticus* because the latter produce a beta-like hemolysis on blood agar and do not produce the characteristic hydrogen sulfide in the butt of a TSI slant. *Listeria monocytogenes* has a characteristic tumbling motility, is usually hemolytic, and ferments salicin and hydrolyzes esculin.

■ **What characteristics do the bacteria, chlamydiae, rickettsia, and mycoplasma share?**

All of these are "bacterial" in characteristics. Each is characterized by the presence of both ribonucleic and deoxyribonucleic acid, binary fission as the method of reproduction, the presence of energy-yielding autonomous metabolism, antibiotic susceptibility, and the presence of ribosomes.

■ **What is BCG?**

BCG or bacille Calmette-Guérin is a vaccine prepared from an attenuated living avirulent strain of *Mycobacterium bovis*. The vaccine is administered intracutaneously and stimulates the production of delayed hypersensitivity and partial immunity to infection with *M. tuberculosis* and *M. bovis*. Individuals who have been vaccinated will convert and maintain a positive tuberculin reaction for many years and during this period are probably adequately protected from tuberculosis. Individuals who are tuberculin positive should not be given BCG.

This procedure has not been universally adopted. It is used in the United States in local areas in which crowding, poverty, or undernourishment prevail or in families in whom exposure to active tuberculosis infection exists. Some countries practice BCG vaccination of the total population and have been able to significantly reduce their incidence of tuberculosis.

■ **What in vivo test may be used to detect hypersensitivity to tuberculin?**

OT (old tuberculin) or PPD (purified protein derivative) are the active preparations. They may be injected intradermally (Mantoux), scratched onto the surface of the skin (Von Pirquet), applied to the skin on a patch of filter paper (Vollmer), pricked 1 to 2 mm into the skin (Heath), or introduced into the skin with a multiple puncture instrument (Tine).

■ **Which stool specimens should be processed without delay for parasites?**

All specimens should be processed without undue delay. However, it is very important to examine promptly if trophozoite movement is to be observed. A dysenteric mucus and blood-tinged stool from a patient infected with *Entamoeba histolytica* is such a specimen. Of course, it is sometimes difficult to guess the etiology of dysentery or severe diarrhea. Bacillary dysentery caused by the shigellae may produce similar specimens and must be promptly processed.

■ **Many parasitic infestations can be diagnosed by the finding of cysts or trophozoites in the stool specimen. Describe the method of laboratory confirmation of trichinosis.**

Trichinosis is acquired upon eating contaminated meat such as pork. The adult forms inhabit the digestive tract of man and produce larval forms that invade the tissues of the same host, without going through an intermediary host. The parasite does not occur in free form in any of its developmental phases and therefore cannot be identified from the stool specimen.

The early laboratory diagnosis is very difficult and is rarely made. During the first few days, adult worms may occasionally be observed by sedimentation of feces. From the end of the first week until the end of larval migration, larva may be demonstrated from the blood of those heavily infected (1 to 2 larva/ml). Biopsy of the encysted larva may be done on the deltoid, biceps, and gastrocnemius muscles. Serologic analysis may serve as an adjunct to clinical diagnosis but is usually not specific enough to be used alone. Positive skin and precipitin tests have about the same specificity but the skin test may be negative in the very light and very heavy infestations.

■ **Differentiate *Taenia solium* from *T. saginata*.**

The larvae of *T. solium* are found in pig (and man) whereas the *T. saginata* is found in cattle and humans. The scolex of *T. solium* is armed with a double row of hooks, the gravid uterus has 5 to 13 branches, and the proglottids are passed in long chains. In contrast, the *T. saginata* scolex is without hooks, the gravid uterus has from 15 to 30 branches, and the proglottids are usually passed singly.

The two cannot be differentiated on the appearance of the egg.

■ **A trophozoite measuring approximately 19μ with ingested red blood cells was seen in a stool specimen. What species might this represent and how would you differentiate between them?**

The size would suggest *Entamoeba coli* or a large race *E. histolytica* from a case of amebic dysentery. Although it is rare for *E. coli* to ingest red blood cells, it nevertheless does happen in patients with persistent bleeding of the colon, during which time the *E. coli* become conditioned to feed on the red cells.

To eliminate this latter possibility, look for two clues. (1) Cysts: Cysts are usually found even in the presence of trophozoites, unless the stool is quite liquid, or are present in an exudate. If no cysts are found, ask for repeat specimens until a cyst-bearing stool is obtained. (2) Look at a fresh stool for the presence of progressive crawling trophozoite motility. The nucleus of *E. coli* trophozoites is visible but a nucleus is not usually seen in trophozoites of *E. histolytica*. If both of these fail, make stained smears for differentiation of the amoeba or induce constipation to obtain stools with cysts.

■ **A pear-shaped (anterior posterior view) and a spoon-shaped (lateral view) trophozoite measuring about 12 to 15μ long with a slow tumbling or fallen-leaf motion was seen in a duodenal aspirate. Name the probable organism and state the clinical significance.**

Giardia lamblia is probably present. Giardiasis is an infestation of the intestinal tract of man occurring primarily in the duodenum and jejunum. Chronic diarrhea is the most common symptom in adults, occasionally coexisting with steatorrhea and malabsorption. Children are more susceptible to giardiasis than adults.

Epigastric pain, vague abdominal discomfort, loss of appetite, fever, weight loss, and symptoms referable to the liver and gallbladder, i.e., jaundice, may be present. However, many people harbor the parasite in an essentially commensal relationship without symptomatology.

■ **A patient recently returned from a malarial zone was found to have fever every fourth day. On examination of the blood smear a mature schizont was seen to contain 6 merozoites. What malarial parasite might this represent and how would you confirm this?**

This suggests *Plasmodium malariae* infection, the cause of quartan malaria. One should also look for other parasites of different maturation. *P. malariae* rarely has more than one parasite per red cell and has coarse pigment granules in the growing trophozoite. The growing schizonts are compact, oval or round, with 2 to 6 chromatin granules and coarse granules or clumps of pigment. The mature schizont has 6 to 12 merozoites forming a single ring or cluster appearing as a rosette or daisy and has the pigment located as a central mass.

■ **What is the exoerythrocytic cycle of malarial parasites?**

This is a schizogonic stage of development of the malarial parasite that takes place in the reticuloendothelial system and other tissues and is characterized by a lack of malarial pigment. It is thought to develop as certain merozoites of the erythrocytic cycle enter tissue cells or as a result of tissue cell invasion by the macromerozoites that were produced earlier during the preerythrocytic stages.

■ *Trypanosoma gambiense* **and** *T. rhodensiense* **cause African sleeping sickness. How could infection with either of these parasites be confirmed in the laboratory?**

The trypanosomes may be demonstrated from lymph node aspirates, blood, or cerebrospinal fluid. In early disease the enlarged lymph node is the best site from which to obtain material; later the organisms may be readily recovered from blood and occasionally from CSF. Direct examination is the best method of demonstrating the parasites, although culture is sometimes beneficial.

In the cover slipped fresh wet blood mount, movement of the parasite causes characteristic movement of the blood cells. If blood smears are prepared, they should be stained in the same manner as for malarial parasites. Blood concentration employing 2% citrate as an anticoagulant and 2% acetic acid as a lysing solution followed by centrifugation has permitted visualization of parasites in light infections. Inoculation of 2 to 10 ml of blood into guinea pigs, mice, or rats may produce a positive infection in a week or so.

■ **What parasite causes visceral leishmaniasis and what is its morphologic form?**

Leishmania donovani appears in man only in the leishmanian form. It is an intracellular, oval, and nonflagellated body found especially in the cells of the reticuloendothelial system but occasionally in small numbers in the blood. When stained with Giemsa or Wright's stain, a large red nucleus and a purple rod-shaped parabasal body are readily seen. Single macrophages may be heavily parasitized with these bodies.

■ **What are viruses?**

Viruses or virons are small infectious agents that are potentially pathogenic in the susceptible host. They contain either deoxyribonucleic or ribonucleic acid, but not both, which is situated in a core covered by a protein sheath or capsid. The capsid is composed of protein subunits that are packed very closely together in either cubical or helical symmetrical patterns. The host cell replicates more of these infectious units from the viral genetic material. Viruses are insensitive to the effects of antibiotics which are effective against bacteria.

■ **What is the basis of classification of viruses?**

Viruses may be classified in many ways. Clinicians classify them according to the clinical disease associated with them. Virologists classify them according to their nucleic acid content, size, morphology, ether sensitivity, heat lability, and pH lability.

■ **Define tropism as it relates to "target organs."**

An early classification based on the affinity for and localization of a virus in specific tissues, i.e., skin by dermotropic, paralysis by neurotropic, pneumonia by pneumotropic, and enteritis by enterotropic virus, was thought to be highly specific. Although tropisms do exist because of specific receptors localized in the tissues, these characteristics are not stable enough for purposes of classification. Many viruses have no specific tissue affinities. The Coxsackie B virus, for example, can infect such diverse tissues as muscle, brain, meninges, subcutaneous fat, pancreas, heart, and pericardium. Thus tropism offers the least reliable of all factors that can be used in the classification of viruses.

■ **What is the significance of antibodies to the Epstein-Barr virus?**

This herpes-like virus was originally observed in cell cultures from the highly malignant Burkitt's lymphoma common in Central and East African children. This virus has been implicated in infectious mononucleosis; all patients with the infectious mononucleosis syndrome who are infected with this virus as well as all patients with Burkitt's lymphoma have demonstrable antibodies to this agent. This antibody is quite distinct from the heterophile antibody.

■ **What are blastospores and what is the method of reproduction in them?**

Blastospores are round to pyriform asexual reproductive units of yeast and yeast-like organisms. Most reproduce by single budding, but *Paracoccidioides braziliensis* characteristically has multiple budding. Daughter buds are usually joined to the parent blastospore with a narrow point of attachment. However, daughter blastospores of *Blastomyces dermatitidis* are attached by a broad base and have a wide pore between them.

■ **What are arthrospores and which fungi possess them?**

Arthrospores are one of three types of thallospores, which are asexual reproductive spores formed from the thallus or mycelium. The arthrospore is formed by segmentation of the hyphae to form rectangular thick-walled cells. *Geotrichum, Oidium* or *Oospora*, and *Coccidioides* reproduce in this manner in culture. In addition, the dermatophytes exhibit this type of sporulation in tissue.

■ **What is a germ tube and how is the phenomenon of germ tube formation used in the clinical laboratory?**

The germ tube is a short filament arising from a blastospore of *Candida*. If the test is carried out in egg albumin, human serum, or some other similar medium at 37° C and is read within 2 hours, it is reported to be quite specific for *Candida albicans*. It is a useful tool for presumptive identification of colonies of *C. albicans* from clinical material. *C. stellatoidea* is reported to have a positive germ tube in 4 but not in 2 hours at 37° C.

■ **Which fungi may appear as "yeast" forms in human tissue?**

Candida, Cryptococcus, Torulopsis, Geotrichum, Sporothrix (Sporotrichum), Blastomyces, Paracoccidioides, Coccidioides, Histoplasma, and *Loboa* appear as "yeast" forms.

■ **What is the usefulness and limitation of a KOH mount of skin scrapings?**

It is useful to digest the keratinized cells and permit the fungal elements to be visualized. One can differentiate between cutaneous dermatophyte infections and those caused by *Candida*. However, all dermatophytes of the genera *Trichophyton, Microsporum,* and *Epidermophyton* produce arthrospores that are identical to one another.

■ **Of what use is a Wood's light?**

A Wood's light is an ultraviolet light with an emission at 3,660 Å. A shaft of hair infected with *Trichophyton schoenleini* will fluoresce a bluish white, and one infected with *Microsporum* species will fluoresce a greenish-yellow when illuminated with this light in a darkened room. This enables the selection of parasitized hair for examination and culture. A 100-watt Blak-Ray lamp or one of comparable intensity is recommended.

■ **Why is an India ink preparation performed and what are the benefits and limitations of the procedure?**

An India ink preparation is a negative capsule stain used to demonstrate encapsulated blastospores of *Cryptococcus neoformans* in cerebrospinal fluid of patients with *C. neoformans* meningitis. A positive finding of fully encapsulated blastospores that are budding is diagnostic. However, only about 50% of patients with *C. neoformans* meningitis have a positive India ink preparation. For this reason, all suspect spinal fluids must be cultured on Sabouraud's or similar media for this organism. One must exercise caution in interpreting the smear inasmuch as a lymphocyte may simulate a *C. neoformans* blastospore with a small capsule.

■ **Identify *Candida albicans*.**

Candida albicans is a yeast-like fungus that is worldwide in distribution. In man it is found readily as part of skin, vaginal, oral, and gut normal flora. Under proper circumstances the organism can cause local infections on the skin and mucous membranes or become systemic and cause lesions in the lung or kidneys or metastatic lesions throughout the body. It is characterized by its ability to form germ tubes in human serum in 2 hours at 37° C, consistently ferment glucose and maltose, and assimilate glucose, maltose, sucrose, galactose, xylose, and trehalose.

■ **How is candidemia best detected?**

Candidemia may be either transient or associated with *Candida* sepsis. In either instance, the most sensitive and rapid method for isolation is to collect blood with Liquoid (SPS or sodium polyanetheol sulfonate) and lyse with Triton X-100 (alkyl phenoxy polyethoxy ethanol) and sodium carbonate and filter onto a membrane with 0.45μ porosity. The filter should be washed with sterile saline and aseptically placed onto the agar surface of some suitable agar in a petri dish. Growth will almost always appear within 24 hours.

■ **What is thrush?**

Thrush is oral candidiasis caused by *Candida albicans* and characterized by discrete or confluent patches of a cream-white to gray pseudomembrane on the tongue, soft palate, or buccal mucosa. It is found more frequently in the newborn, who is probably contaminated in the birth canal, and in those who are aged, have a debilitating disease, are on broad-spectrum antibiotics, or are diabetic.

■ **What parasite does the tissue form of *Histoplasma capsulatum* resemble and how can it be differentiated?**

The intracellular forms of *H. capsulatum* are small spherical or ovoid bodies in histiocytes measuring 1 to 5μ in diameter and under low magnification on H&E stain resemble *Leishmania*. If the material is well fixed and viewed under high power magnification, the kinetoplast of the *Leishmania* should be visible. Any of the special fungus stains such as Gridley, Periodic Acid-Schiff, or Gomori methenamine silver will stain the *Histoplasma* fungus but will not stain the *Leishmania* parasites.

■ **What fungi are characterized by producing one morphologic form in tissue and a very dissimilar form on culture and are thus designated as diphasic?**

Blastomyces dermatitidis, Coccidioides immitis, Histoplasma capsulatum, Sporothrix (Sporotrichum) schenckii, and *Paracoccidioides braziliensis* are diphasic fungi.

■ **Describe the appearance of *Coccidioides immitis* in tissue.**

The majority of organisms in tissue resemble the nonbudding forms of *Blastomyces dermatitidis* or *Paracoccidioides braziliensis*. They have thick double-contoured walls and may vary from 2 to 200μ in diameter. The material stains in an irregular fashion in the young developing spherule, but as it becomes a more mature spherule it is found to contain many endospores or sporangiospores. The histologic picture will vary from an early pyogenic reaction similar to the response to bacteria, to a granulomatous response of histiocytic exudate and giant cells resulting from reaction to the sporangium.

■ **What similarities exist in the tissue response among *Mycobacterium tuberculosis* and the various systemic fungi?**

A very important reaction in tuberculosis is related to cell-mediated hypersensitivity. The giant cells, tubercle formation, and other granulomatous reactions are reactions to the tuberculoprotein. In like manner, granulomatous reactions or the hypersensitivity components are frequently the most prominent aspect of systemic fungus infections.

■ **What are antibodies?**

Antibodies are globulin protein molecules (immunoglobulins) formed in a susceptible host as a result of stimulation with an antigen (immunogen). They characteristically react specifically with the related antigen in some demonstrable manner.

■ **What is the generally accepted theory of antibody formation?**

The selective theory, advanced by Sir McFarland Burnet, holds that the information required for the synthesis of different antibodies already resides in the genetic apparatus prior to exposure to the antigen or immunogen. Upon contact between the immunogen and the proper cell, the gene which is responsible for coding for a specific antibody protein is selected and "turned on." Through transcription and translation of the appropriate messenger RNA, specific peptide (immunoglobulin) chains, along with their corresponding individual primary amino acid sequences, are synthesized. As a result of this sequence, the chains fold spontaneously into a preferred globular configuration that has the specific antigen or immunogen combining sites.

■ **What is the difference between "affinity" and "avidity" as applied to antigen-antibody reactions?**

The term "affinity" is used to describe the equilibrium for the reaction between an antigen binding site on the antibody and the determinant on the immunogen (i.e., monovalent hapten), whereas the term "avidity" is applied to the reaction between whole molecules of antigen and immunogen where the valency of the reactants becomes involved.

■ **What is an anamnestic response?**

This secondary, or memory, response is observed upon second exposure to an antigen. Antibodies or immunocompetent cells are produced more rapidly and the latent period is shortened or nonexistent. Antibody levels are higher and persist longer than in the primary response. IgG is the principal antibody produced.

■ **What bioactive products are produced by the complement sequence?**

C1,4 results in the neutralization of herpes simplex viruses that have been sensitized by IgM antibody.

C1,4,2 is thought to produce a kinin-like material that will contract smooth muscle and cause increased vascular permeability. This kinin-like material is resistant to the antihistamine drugs.

C3b, attached to a red blood cell, may lead to rapid cell destruction, recognized as autoimmune hemolytic disorder. On the surface of red cells, platelets, or leukocytes C3b will bring out immune adherence. This is a phenomenon in which each cell will cause attachment or adherence to normal RBC's with resulting agglutination in vitro.

C3a biotoxic activities include anaphylatoxin, which causes contraction of smooth muscle, release of histamine from mast cells and increased vascular permeability, and a second action of induction of leukocyte chemotaxis or the attraction of neutrophilic granulocytes in a unidirectional manner.

C5a, in an analogus manner to C3a, has anaphylatoxic and chemotactic properties for granulocytes. It is thought that C5b is important in some phagocytic systems.

C5,6,7, or activated trimolecular complex, has chemotactic activity for neutrophiles.

It is known that if C8 and C9 react with the earlier portion of the complement sequence in proximity to a cell surface, a cytotoxic alteration of the membrane occurs, resulting in the loss of the functional integrity of the cells and the loss of cellular constituents. Such cells are irreversibly damaged.

■ **What are complement fixation tests?**

Complement fixation tests, complement-dependent lytic reactions, are in vitro manifestations of antigen-antibody interaction. These reactions form the basis for laboratory tests used in the detection and identification of antigens and antibodies involved in disease processes.

■ **Where does complement react with the immunoglobulin molecule?**

Complement reacts with the Fc portion of the antibody molecule. Different immunoglobulin classes have different Fc structures and not all will bind complement. This characteristic is shared only with IgM and IgG. There are even differences among the various subclasses of IgG: IgG_1 and IgG_3 fix complement well, IgG_2 less so, and IgG_4 poorly if at all. The Clq molecule, which is linked in a trimolecular complex to Clr and Cls, is polyvalent and needs to combine with at least two Fc sites for activation. This presents no problem with the pentavalent IgM molecule, because several Fc regions are readily available within one molecule. However, IgG can fix complement when two or more molecules are bound to closely adjacent sites on the antigen.

■ **What is the significance of IgM in the infectious process?**

IgM is the immunoglobulin class which has the greatest antibacterial activity. IgM is formed early in the immune response and serves as an opsonin, promoting phagocytosis. It immobilizes bacteria by agglutination and causes lysis by efficient activation of complement.

■ **What are reagins?**

Reagins are IgE antibodies which mediate "allergic" or "atopic" states. They comprise a very small part (0.002%) of the total serum immunoglobulin. There is a cytophilic affinity of the Fc portion of IgE (ϵ-chain) and the membrane of mast cells, neutrophils, and basophils. IgE can sensitize these cells to allergens and upon subsequent contact with the allergen will immediately undergo degranulation with the release of vasoactive substances such as histamine and histamine-like substances.

■ **What is transfer factor?**

Transfer factor is a dialyzable polypeptide extracted from human lymphocytes and is capable of transferring cell-mediated immunity to a number of antigens including tuberculin and diphtheria toxoid. Its precise mode of action is unknown.

■ **What is lymphotoxin (LT)?**

Lymphotoxin is a heat-stable substance of about 80,000 to 150,000 molecular weight which has been liberated from specifically sensitized lymphocytes, as well as lymphocytes stimulated by nonspecific stimulators, such as phytohemagglutinin (PHA). This substance seemingly inhibits the capacity of cells to undergo division and is associated with target cell injury.

■ **How is it thought that the immune response system plays a role in the pathogenesis of poststreptococcal glomerulonephritis?**

Following an upper respiratory tract infection with certain types of Group A *Streptococcus pyogenes,* antistreptococcal antibodies are formed. These antibodies complex with circulating streptococcal antigens and are filtered out by the renal glomeruli and deposited in the Bowman's space aspect of the capillary basement membrane. Subsequent binding of complement initiates acute inflammation of the glomeruli with increased glomerular permeability, leading to the leakage of proteins and cells into the urine.

Immunofluorescent procedures demonstrate "lumpy-bumpy" deposits of IgG and complement on the outside of the glomerular basement membrane.

■ **What two dissimilar populations of small lymphocytes are present and to what phase of the immune response are they related?**

T-lymphocytes are processed by or are in some way dependent upon the thymus. These small lymphocytes are responsible for cell-mediated hypersensitivity, i.e., tuberculin hypersensitivity.

B-lymphocytes are bursa dependent, at least as demonstrated in the chicken, and are concerned with the synthesis of circulating antibody. In man and other mammals, no specific anatomic structure such as the bursa of Fabricius has been found. However, gut-associated lymphoid tissue such as the tonsil, Peyer's patches, and appendix are thought to serve this purpose.

■ **Can a primary T-cell deficiency predispose an individual to bacterial infection?**

We are aware that the T-cell small lymphocytes are related to cell-mediated hypersensitivity and the ability to handle viral infections. However, the ability to handle bacteria that have a hypersensitivity component depends upon the presence of a functional T-cell system. Thus even the administration of the attenuated BCG (bacille Calmette Guérin, or attenuated *Mycobacterium bovis*) can be devastating to a child with primary T-cell deficiency.

■ **How would a primary B-cell deficiency manifest itself in a child?**

The child would be expected to have normal cell-mediated immune responses and would have the ability to handle viral infections such as measles and smallpox readily.

However, inasmuch as the humoral response would be depressed, the production of specific immunoglobulins would be grossly depressed and the child would be subject to repeated infection with pyogenic bacteria, such as *Staphylococcus aureus, Streptococcus pyogenes, S. pneumoniae, Neisseria meningitidis,* and *Haemophilus influenzae.* In addition, *Candida albicans,* a fungus, and *Pneumocystis carinii,* a protozoan, could cause severe infections. Histologically, there would be few lymphoid follicles or plasma cells present in lymph node biopsies.

■ **Can an antibody molecule react with the Fab and Fc portions at the same time?**

Yes. In the classic reaction the Fab portion of the immunoglobulin combines with the immunogen or homologous antigen. However, antibody to the class of immunoglobulin or its heavy chain could react with the Fc portion. Thus we would react antigen versus antibody in a classic agar gel precipitation reaction and then react radioactive tagged antibody to the different heavy chains to discover the class of antibody of immunoglobulin that was entering into the reaction.

■ **How do the various serologic tests compare in sensitivity when measuring antibody nitrogen of high avidity antibody?**

The precipitin and immunoelectrophoresis tests are the least sensitive, requiring 3 to 20 mg Ab N/ml per test. Double diffusion in agar gel is slightly more sensitive, requiring 0.2 to 1.0 mg Ab N/ml per test. At the other end of the spectrum, the virus neutralization and bactericidal test require only 1×10^{-4} to 1×10^{-5} mg Ab N. Almost as sensitive is the radioimmunoassay and antigen-combining globulin technique (Farr) of 1×10^{-3} to 1×10^{-4} mg.

The intermediate tests are complement-fixation, 0.01 to 0.1; radial immunodiffusion, 0.008 to 0.025; bacterial agglutination, 0.01; hemolysis, 0.001 to 0.03; passive hemagglutination, 0.005; and antitoxin neutralization, 0.003 mg Ab N/ml per test.

The in vivo passive cutaneous anaphylaxis test requires 0.003 mg Ab N. Accordingly, one must select the test with the proper sensitivity if one wishes to perform serologic quantitation of antibody.

■ **What is the rheumatoid factor and what is its clinical significance?**

The rheumatoid factor is a macroglobulin or immunoglobulin belonging to the IgM class which is found primarily in the alpha globulin, although to some extent it may be found in the beta fraction of serum. It may be found in the serum of rheumatoid arthritis and systemic lupus erythematosus patients even though they may lack the clinical manifestations of the disease. Trauma, fatigue, and emotional factors have also been incriminated as possible etiologic and/or precipitating factors. The factor agglutinates a variety of suspended particles including hemolytic streptococci, sheep red blood cells sensitized with antisheep erythrocyte rabbit serum, latex, and bentonite suspensions.

Significant titers for rheumatoid arthritis vary with the test procedure. For the sheep cell agglutinin it is 232; bentonite, 32; and latex, 20. The hemagglutinin reaction with sensitized sheep erythrocytes, although positive in up to 90% of cases of rheumatoid arthritis, is also positive in 15 to 25% of SLE, an occasional case of sarcoidosis, syphilis, scleroderma, and 1 to 4% of normal human sera.

■ **How does cross reactivity influence the interpretation of immunodiagnostic tests for unknown fevers?**

The febrile agglutination tests are used to detect antibodies to various bacteria, i.e., *Salmonella, Brucella, Francisella tularensis,* and *Rickettsia.* Inasmuch as many of the *Salmonella* antigens are shared with various members of the genus and family, there will be cross agglutination whenever this occurs. However, if a battery of antigens is used, the agglutination will occur quicker and will be stronger with the homologous antigen than with the minor or cross reacting one.

Of course, cross reaction is the basis of the detection of *Rickettsia* antibodies with suspensions of various *Proteus* strains in the Weil-Felix reaction. In addition, a good history is important to evaluate the agglutination reactions with *Brucella* and *Francisella tularensis* antigens.

■ **Define and discuss the clinical significance of the C-reactive protein.**

The C-reactive protein is an abnormal protein that appears in the blood of patients with acute inflammatory reactions but is absent in healthy individuals. It is an alpha globulin whose production is stimulated by various bacterial infections, pyrogenic agents, or products of injured tissue. It is predictably present in rheumatic activity and serves as a sensitive and reliable indicator of inflammatory activity. Conversely, the disappearance of the C-reactive protein reflects effective treatment or spontaneous remission.

■ **What is the Weil-Felix test?**

The Weil-Felix test is an agglutination procedure used to detect antibodies to various rickettsia belonging to the genus *Rickettsia* but not the genus *Coxiella*. The antigen used in this test is one of several strains of *Proteus* designated OX-19, OX-2, and OX-K. Although low titers of agglutinins may be found in an infection with *Proteus*, titers of several hundred are found with the typhus fevers and Rocky Mountain spotted fever.

■ **What is the significance of cold agglutinins or cold reacting antibodies?**

Antibodies for human type O erythrocytes active at 0 to 10° C may be found in a variety of acute infections such as *Mycoplasma pneumoniae*, infectious mononucleosis, trypanosomiasis, and congenital cytomegalovirus infection. The common use of this test is in the patient with primary atypical pneumonia (PAP) caused by *M. pneumoniae*. Although cold agglutinins appear in only about 50% of the mild cases of infectious mononucleosis, they are present in greater percentage and are found in higher titer in severe cases.

■ **What are Forssman antibodies?**

Forssman antibodies belong to the class of heterophile antibodies. Immunization of rabbits with guinea pig tissues stimulates the production of antibodies that agglutinate sheep red blood cells. These nonspecies-specific antibodies are Forssman antibodies.

■ **What relationship do the heterophile antibodies have to infectious mononucleosis?**

Antisheep or heterophile agglutinins may be found in low titer in normal individuals. During infectious mononucleosis, the heterophile antibody titer may increase to 224 or greater. This, coupled with characteristic clinical symptomatology, is presumptive evidence of this disease.

Heterophile antibodies may be observed in serum sickness. To differentiate among these three heterophile antibodies, the serum should be adsorbed with guinea pig extract to remove the agglutinins of serum sickness or the naturally occurring heterophile antibody. The heterophile antibody of infectious mononucleosis is not removed by guinea pig adsorption but is removed by ox cell adsorption.

■ **What serologic tests can be used to evaluate the patient for recent streptococcal infection?**

Antistreptolysin O, antihyaluronidase, and antideoxyribonuclease tests are the tests of choice.

■ **How does immunization affect the typhoid O and H antibodies in the Widal test?**

Immunization causes a rise in the H agglutinins. However, active infection causes an early rise of O agglutinins followed by H agglutinins, which persist longer. H agglutinins only would suggest a previous infection or immunization, whereas positive reactions involving the O antigens would be more suggestive of an active infection.

■ **Discuss the laboratory aids available to assist in the diagnosis of brucellosis.**

A positive culture is the most reliable indicator of brucellosis. The next most reliable test is the agglutinin test. Titers of 320 or greater are usually found in the active case. A fourfold increase in titer is necessary for a serologic diagnosis. However, even some patients with a positive blood culture have low titers of antibodies or occasionally are negative altogether. The presence of incomplete and blocking antibodies must be considered. The prozone phenomenon has been demonstrated up to titers of 400, but this can be minimized by use of a 5% NaCl solution as the diluent. The incomplete antibodies can be detected with Coomb's serum.

■ **What is the principle of the VDRL slide test for syphilis?**

The VDRL antigen is composed of purified cardiolipin and lecithin from beef heart with cholesterol added to increase the antigen's effective reacting surface. Reagin from syphilis, or any other disease which produces reagin, produces dispersion of the cardiolipin lecithin antigen that is observed as a visible flocculation.

■ **What is the usefulness of the FTA-ABS test in evaluating the questionable syphilitic patient?**

The FTA-ABS is an indirect fluorescent antibody test devised to detect antibodies in the patient's serum which are specific for the spirochete *Treponema pallidum*. In the procedure, the nonspecific reacting substances in the serum are removed by a sorbent prepared from a sonicate of the nonpathogenic Reiter treponeme. Thus, antibodies "specific" for the *T. pallidum* remain in the serum. Although a rare serum will still exhibit fluorescence in the absence of syphilis, the test remains one of the most reliable and easily performed of current syphilis serologic procedures.

The FTA-ABS test becomes reactive about as quickly as the reagin tests (i.e., VDRL, RPR, etc.) in primary syphilis, 3 to 4 weeks, but remains reactive even after effective therapy. Thus, the FTA-ABS is the test to be used for confirmation of syphilis or to rule out syphilis when the commonly used screening tests detect nonsyphilitic reagin.

■ **When would a spinal fluid VDRL examination be indicated?**

When there is a suspicion of neurosyphilis. False positive reactions in the CSF are very rare. The presence of reagin in the CSF is the only finding which is highly indicative and a reliable indicator of present or past neurosyphilis. A diagnosis of latent syphilis can be confirmed only if asymptomatic neurosyphilis is ruled out with a negative reagin test of the CSF.

■ **How does the RPR card test compare with other serologic tests for syphilis?**

The RPR or rapid plasma reagin card test has the same significance as any other reagin test when reactive or nonreactive. Its sensitivity and specificity are comparable to those of the VDRL. However, the antigen in the RPR test is much more stable than the VDRL and is the test to be preferred when experts trained in the preparation of the VDRL antigen of standard reactivity are not found. This includes developing countries, field laboratories, small laboratories which perform only occasional serologic tests for syphilis, and indeed even many of the serologic units in some larger hospitals.

■ **Describe the principle of the hemagglutination-inhibition test and its diagnostic importance.**

Certain viruses have the ability to agglutinate erythrocytes from various species. This activity can be inhibited by specific antibody. Thus antibodies in serum against viruses such as influenza, measles, and rubella can be detected by serum's ability to inhibit the viral hemagglutinating activity.

■ **What is counterimmunoelectrophoresis? What is its most common laboratory application?**

Counterimmunoelectrophoresis is a modification of immunoelectrophoresis in which antigen and antibody are driven toward each other by an electrical field. This speeds the reaction and increases its sensitivity. This procedure is most commonly used to detect hepatitis associated antigen (HAA).

■ **Describe the principle of radial immunodiffusion. For what is this technique used?**

Specific antisera are incorporated into an agar gel for unknown sera and known standards. A known amount of serum is placed in the wells, and plates are incubated in a moist chamber at room temperature. The proteins diffuse from the wells into the gel. The specific antigen combines with the antibody in the gel, forming a circular precipitation line. The diameter of this circle is proportional to the concentration of antigen in the serum.

This procedure may be used to quantitate serum components such as immunoglobulins, transferrin, complement C3, and alpha-1 antitrypsin.

■ **What abnormality in serum immunoglobulins is often associated with helminth infection?**

Increased levels of IgE are commonly observed in patients with parasitic diseases. Other allergic manifestations such as urticaria, asthma, and rashes also characterize these diseases. It is thought that IgE may function as a local defense against parasitic disease.

CHAPTER 7

Instrumentation and quality control

JOHN D. REEVES

■ **Distinguish between photometer, colorimeter, and spectrophotometer.**

The photometer is any instrument that measures the intensity of a beam of light. A colorimeter, in the clinical laboratory, specifically refers to the instrument used to measure the intensity of colored light. It is understood that the color (range of wavelengths) used is selected by some sort of filter, thus the alternate designation of filter photometer. A spectrophotometer also measures light intensity; but, with the addition of a device to disperse the source light into a continuous spectrum, it permits the selection of any desired wavelength in the available range and provides improved control over the range of adjacent wavelengths included in the beam produced.

■ **What is monochromatic light and what devices can be used to produce it?**

Monochromatic light literally means "light of one color." In spectrophotometry, we would like to consider true monochromatic light to be defined as light radiation of a single wavelength, although what a monochromator provides in practice is always a range of wavelengths on both sides of the desired one. The average spectral width of this range expressed in units of wavelengths is the band pass; this is the characteristic which distinguishes different monochromator systems.

The major monochromating devices are the following. (1) The colored filter, usually glass, absorbs some portions of the electro-

118

magnetic spectrum and transmits others. Light energy is absorbed by dye compounds in the glass and is ultimately dissipated as heat. The band pass is quite wide, perhaps 35 to 50 nm or greater. (2) The interference filter utilizes the wave character of light to enhance the intensity of the desired wavelength by constructive interference and eliminates other wavelengths by destructive interference and reflection. Band pass can be limited to 10 to 20 nm with these filters. (3) A prism disperses white light into a continuous spectrum of colors based on small differences in refractive index for different wavelengths of light, red light having a lower refractive index than the shorter violet light. Any band of wavelengths can be isolated by projecting this spectrum onto the exit slit. The band pass can be limited to a few nanometers, although this becomes increasingly difficult toward the long wave regions where the nonlinear dispersion of the prism results in a crowded spectrum. (4) The most common dispersing device used today, particularly in the lower cost spectrophotometers for clinical laboratory applications, is the diffraction grating. It is generally manufactured as a replica grating. Gratings may be either transmission or reflectance type, although both are basically pieces of optical glass with very closely spaced precision parallel grooves (approximately 15,000 per inch). The spectrum is produced by interference resulting from small path differences between light waves as they are scattered by the narrow grooves. The grating has two advantages over the prism as a dispersing device: (a) it produces a linear spectrum, therefore maintaining a constant band pass is simple; (b) it can be used in the regions of the spectrum where light energy is absorbed by glass prisms (UV and IR).

■ **Define nominal wavelength and band pass width.**

The nominal wavelength is the one which is read off the selection dial of the spectrophotometer and is located in the center of the spectral segment of wavelengths which actually pass through the exit slit to form the final beam of monochromatic light. In the spectrophotometer the band pass depends on the design of the monochromator but is essentially equivalent to the spectral width (in nanometers) of the exit slit. For a filter, the true definition of band pass is more explanatory: the range of wavelengths between the two points where transmission intensity is one-half that of the transmission peak (which occurs at the nominal wavelength).

■ **Describe four different types of photodetectors.**

(1) The photovoltaic cell, formerly referred to as a barrier layer cell, is commonly constructed of a plate of metal (e.g., iron) covered with a thin layer of a photosensitive semiconductor material (e.g., selenium). The photosensitive layer emits electrons in direct proportion to the intensity of the light impinging on it. The current produced can be measured directly with a galvanometer and is reasonably linear with respect to the light intensity. The spectral sensitivity of this device resembles that of the human eye (400 to 800 nm) and is most sensitive to light of about 550 nm. (2) The photoemissive tube consists of two electrodes sealed in an evacuated glass envelope. The cathode is coated with a photosensitive mixture which emits electrons when struck by light radiation. The anode is maintained at a high positive potential and attracts the released electrons, resulting in a flow of photocurrent through the tube. (3) The photomultiplier tube uses the same principle as the photoemissive tube but uses a series of additional electrodes (dynodes) to internally amplify the photosignal before it leaves the tube. The original electrons from the photocathode are accelerated through a series of dynodes, each maintained at a higher positive potential than the last and each coated with a material that will easily release electrons. The photocurrent increases geometrically through the cascade, resulting in a high output signal for a very low-level original input of radiant energy. (4) Junction photodiodes and phototransistors are light-sensitive semiconductor devices coming into use in some clinical laboratory equipment. These are both generally operated as photoconductive type devices. They increase their ability to conduct reverse current when light is focused on the semiconductor junction (the base of the transistor). These both require an external power source and exhibit dark current like phototubes.

■ **List several different types of readout devices used in laboratory instruments.**

Some readout devices are: (1) meter, (2) mechanical digital counter, (3) digital vacuum tubes, (4) LED (light emitting diodes), (5) CRT (cathode ray tubes), (6) line printers, (7) strip chart recorders, and (8) liquid crystal digital readout.

■ **What is the significance of the combined laws referred to as Beer's law?**

Beer's law is fundamental to quantitative absorption photometry. It relates the reduction of radiant power (intensity) of a beam of monochromatic light to the concentration of a sample solute of interest. The law is variously stated as:

$$\left\{ \log \frac{I_o}{I} \text{ or } \log \frac{1}{T} \text{ or } 2\text{-log } \%T \text{ or } A \right\} = abc$$

where

I_o = Intensity of the light incident on the sample
I = Intensity of the light transmitted through the sample
T = Transmittance (a defined term equal to $\frac{I}{I_o}$)

$\%T = T \times 100$

A = Absorbance (a defined term equal to $\log \frac{1}{T}$)

a = Absorptivity (a constant, characteristic of the absorbing specie)
b = Thickness of the absorbing solution (optical light path)
c = Concentration of the absorbing specie in the light path

Note that absorbance has been defined so as to make things easier to work with since it is a linear function with respect to concentration. Calibration curves with concentration plotted against absorbance produce a straight line on graph paper with rectangular coordinates. The graphical plot of T or $\%T$ versus concentration produces an exponential curve on rectangular coordinates, although a straight line can be obtained by plotting log $\%T$ versus concentration (semilog chart paper simplifies handling the log values). The practical application of Beer's law includes some very important assumptions about the nature of the absorbing specie and the conditions under which the analysis is made. These can be directly evaluated by experimentally determining the relationship between absorbance and concentration for the system of interest. One of the most important assumptions is that one is using a truly monochromatic light source. As a wider band pass is employed, deviations from the predicted linear relationship become more apparent. However, useful quantitative results may still be obtained with the careful use of a standard curve and adequate quality control.

■ **Describe the rationale for the selection of the best wavelength for quantitative determinations by absorption spectrophotometry.**

The spectral absorption curve for the compound of interest will indicate the regions of the spectrum where absorbance is maximal as well as minimal. The wavelengths of these absorption peaks are characteristic of the structure of the compound and in the visible and ultraviolet regions they are related to the energy transitions of valence electrons. For the greatest quantitative sensitivity (greatest absorbance change per unit of concentration) the wavelength of greatest absorption is chosen. This selection would be tempered by the consideration of potential measurement errors which are introduced either by variations in instrument use (e.g., reproducing wavelength settings) or the presence of interfering compounds that absorb in the same region. A broad absorption peak may be preferable to a narrow one of slightly greater height, particularly for wide band pass instruments. Occasionally a wavelength on the shoulder of the absorption peak may be used to intentionally reduce the sensitivity of the method as a compromise to gain an increased range of linearity on the standard curve. The pitfall in this technique is the necessity for accurate wavelength settings in order to retain reproducibility in the results. In practice, the problem can be circumvented by including appropriate standards with each analysis.

■ **What is dark current?**

When two electrodes of a photodetector are maintained at different electrical potentials (i.e., have a voltage across them), they tend to "leak" electrons, producing a small flow of current even in the absence of stimulating light. Since this current does not represent the measurement of light radiation, it would introduce an error if it were added to the true photocurrent; therefore it is neutralized by a variable resistance (the zero adjustment).

■ **What instrument component failures would produce instability at zero %T in the spectrophotometer? At 100%T?**

Instability (fluctuation) at zero suggests a weak or defective amplifier tube. Sustained drifting (in one direction) may implicate the power supply. Instability at 100%T, but not at zero, suggests an unstable light source (or power supply) or a noisy or failing photodetector.

■ **What would you conclude from the inability to set 100%T at the lower extreme of the visible region (tungsten light source)?**

The tungsten lamp emits only a small amount of radiation in the violet portion of the spectrum, its peak emission being in the IR. Consequently the detector sensitivity, amplifier gain, and light source emission must all be in respectable condition for adequate operation at this end of the spectrum. This problem most likely indicates that an amplifier tube is aging or that the lamp has deteriorated.

■ **How can the accuracy of the spectrophotometer's wavelength calibration be verified?**

Although the exact procedure depends on the capability of the instrument in question, the general philosophy is the same. Since the emission line spectra of some lamps (e.g., hydrogen, deuterium, helium) and the absorption spectra of pure compounds (didymium and holmium oxide) are characteristic of the material, an instrument in calibration should be able to confirm these established wavelength peaks. Generally a prism instrument should be checked at several points since the prism dispersion is not linear, although two points may be adequate for a grating instrument. Wide band pass instruments commonly used in routine colorimetric methods can be checked with any reproducible colored solution with a characteristic absorption peak (e.g., cobalt chloride, nickel sulfate).

■ **What is an isosbestic point?**

Since the absorption spectrum of a compound is intimately related to the structure of its molecule, it is not surprising that different forms of the same compound will have absorption peaks at different wavelengths. The isosbestic point is a wavelength where all equilibrium forms of the molecule have the same absorptivity (absorbance per unit of concentration), so quantitative measurements using this wavelength will be independent of the changes in the chemical equilibrium. This principle is used in several hemoglobinometers (using 548.5 nm) and oximeters on the market.

■ **What is the difference between a total consumption burner and a premix type?**

The total consumption burner aspirates sample directly into the base of the flame. The oxidant enters the flame at high velocity through a path concentric to that of the sample capillary. The high velocity of the oxidant produces an area of reduced pressure over the capillary. All of the sample drawn into the capillary by the partial vacuum is sheared into fine droplets and consumed in the flame. In the premix configuration, the stream of oxidant passes perpendicularly over the sample capillary and throws the resulting mist against the wall of the atomizer chamber. Most of the droplets flow down the wall and out the waste drain. The remaining finest droplets are combined with the fuel in the upper part of the chamber before the final mixture is injected into the burner. Most recent atomizer-burners are of the premix configuration.

■ **What is the internal standard technique in flame photometry and why is lithium the most common choice?**

In theory, the emission of light in the flame is directly proportional to the concentration of the element in the flame. In practice, several factors modify this ideal relationship and result in differing emission values for the same amount of sample. The internal standard technique incorporates a known constant amount of the standard element in the diluent. The diluent is used for all samples and calibrating solutions. The instrument simultaneously monitors the emission of the standard and each test element through separate photodetectors and calculates the sample concentrations on the basis of electronic comparison with the standard.

Lithium is chosen as the standard for sodium and potassium determinations for two reasons: (1) lithium emission characteristics are sufficiently similar to those of sodium and potassium so that conditions which would produce variations in emission of the test elements would produce similar changes in the lithium emission; (2) lithium is normally a trace element in human tissues and does not present interference. Current use of lithium salts in psychiatric therapy has modified the second condition and generated a clinical demand for lithium determinations since lithium is toxic above about 2 mEq/L in serum. Several recent flame photometers are equipped for lithium determinations and use potassium as the internal standard.

■ **Distinguish the principles of flame emission and atomic absorption photometry.**

When a solution is evaporated in a flame, the salt crystals are vaporized and the cations reduced to their neutral electronic state. The electrons of the neutral atom can be excited to higher energy states by absorbing specific amounts of energy. In flame photometry this absorbed energy comes from the heat of the flame. When these unstable excited electrons return to their original ground state, they emit exactly the same quantity of energy that was required to reach the excited condition. In both techniques the central unifying concept is that a given electronic transition requires a very specific quanta of energy to raise the energy state, and the transition downward liberates the same quantity of energy. Light can be the form of energy involved in these transitions. The quantity of energy in a beam of light is inversely related to the wavelength. Therefore a given electronic transition always involves the same wavelength of light. Flame emission photometry quantitates the number of atoms present in the flame as a function of the light emitted by the small percentage of atoms which become excited and return to ground state. Atomic absorption measures the much more numerous neutral atoms in the flame as a function of their ability to absorb light energy. The wavelength of light absorbed is identical to that emitted in the case of flame photometry since the identical electronic transition is involved. In atomic absorption, whether or not the excited atom returns to ground state and emits light is unimportant.

■ **List the basic components of a simple fluorometer.**

The basic components of a simple fluorometer are: (1) a source of exciting radiation—generally in the UV region; (2) a primary monochromator to isolate the exciting wavelength—an absorption filter is the simplest; (3) a cuvette to hold the sample; (4) a secondary monochromator to isolate the wavelength of fluorescence emission, while blocking any stray radiation from the exciting beam; (5) a photodetector to measure the fluorescence emission; usually a photomultiplier since the intensity of fluorescence is quite low (NOTE: The path of exciting radiation and the path from the sample to the detector are commonly placed perpendicular to avoid detecting interfering emission of the source); and (6) a readout system.

■ **What is a glass electrode and how does it measure pH?**

The glass electrode for pH measurement consists of an internal reference electrode (e.g., silver/silver chloride) submerged in a solution of known pH and enclosed in a glass bulb of special pH-sensitive glass. The sensitive glass is usually fused to a barrel of high resistance glass which is not pH-sensitive in order to avoid measurement errors from varying depths of immersion. The special glass develops a potential difference between its two surfaces which is proportional to the difference between the pH values of the test solution and the internal solution. The potential must be measured using a second reference electrode immersed in the test solution and an electronic voltmeter with very high input impedance.

■ **Describe two common types of reference electrodes for pH measurement.**

Two reference electrodes are: (1) calomel (mercury chloride) electrode—consists of an inert lead-in wire (e.g., platinum) in contact with a paste of mercury and mercury chloride and surrounded by a solution of KCl saturated with calomel; and (2) silver/silver chloride electrode—consists of a metallic silver wire coated with a layer of silver chloride and surrounded by a solution of KCl saturated with silver chloride. In both cases, electrical contact with the test solution is accomplished by a salt bridge of KCl.

■ **How does the Severinghaus CO_2 electrode measure P_{CO_2}?**

The CO_2 electrode consists of a combination pH electrode immersed in a buffer solution of $KHCO_3$ and covered with a gas-permeable membrane (e.g., Teflon). Carbon dioxide gas diffuses across the membrane at a rate proportional to its partial pressure in the sample. The interaction of CO_2 (as carbonic acid) and $KHCO_3$ results in a change in pH which can be measured directly with the pH electrode and electronically related to the P_{CO_2}.

■ **How does a P_{O_2} electrode work?**

The principle is based on the technique of polarography. The electrode consists of a platinum cathode and a tubular silver anode which are electrically connected by an electrolyte filling solution at their tips. The entire sensing tip is covered with a gas-permeable membrane. The electrodes are maintained at a constant potential of about 0.8 V. The oxygen diffuses across the membrane at a rate proportional to its partial pressure in the sample and is reduced at the cathode. The oxidation product, silver oxide, is subsequently formed at the silver anode. The small current produced as a result of this exchange of electrons is measured by an electrometer against a reference electrode and can be electronically related to the P_{O_2}.

■ **What does the slope control on a pH meter actually adjust?**

The pH meter measures pH as a function of the potential difference (voltage) between the two electrodes. If the actual millivolt response of the system is plotted against the pH of known buffers, the slope of the line produced represents the millivolt change per pH unit. The slope control adjusts this response to the theoretical (Nernst) value of 59.16 mv/pH unit at 25° C. Since the response is linear, the slope can be set by calibrating the meter at any second pH value (e.g., pH 4.01) after calibration at mid-range (i.e., pH 7.0).

■ **Why are both voltage and current levels of interest in electro-phoresis?**

Electrophoresis separates proteins on the basis of their differences in net electrical charge. The rate of migration in an electric field is directly related to the applied voltage. Higher voltages produce faster separations and generally better resolution. The amount of current which flows in the system is a significant indication of the amount of heat that is generated and must be successfully dissipated to avoid distortions of pattern, denaturation of protein, or drying of the support medium. High current should be avoided because the power (heat) dissipation increases as the square of the current.

■ **What is the principle of the Coulter Company's cell counting devices?**

A suitable dilution of cells is prepared in an electrolyte solution and a known volume of the dilution is drawn through an aperture of small diameter (e.g., 100μ). A constant regulated current is maintained between two platinum electrodes placed on either side of the electrolyte filled aperture. The cells are poor electrical conductors themselves but they displace their volume of electrolyte as they pass through the aperture. The increased resistance (or decreased conductivity) to current flow results in a momentary pulse representing the increased voltage drop across the aperture as the cell passes through the orifice. The instrument recognizes and counts the cells as electrical pulses. The instrument can electronically discriminate cells of a selected size since the pulse size is directly proportional to the cell size. Coincidence losses caused by simultaneous passage of more than one cell through the aperture can be predicted statistically and thus corrected according to the total number of cells counted in the aliquot.

■ **What is the function of the mercury manometer in the Coulter counter?**

The mercury column is unbalanced when vacuum is momentarily applied to one end. As it returns to its equilibrium position, it syphons the diluted cell suspension through the aperture at a uniform rate. The mercury, being electrically conductive, is also used as a switching device to control the counting section of the instrument. Three electrodes (start, stop, and common) are implanted in the wall of the mercury-filled manometer tubing in contact with the mercury. The volume displaced by the mercury between the start and stop signals is exactly 0.5 ml. The cell suspension is drawn through the aperture during the entire time the mercury column is in motion, but the instrument counts only the cells in the aliquot predetermined by the position of the start and stop electrodes.

■ **What is another principle used in automated cell counting devices?**

Generally, it involves an optical system, although there are considerable variations. The cell suspension is passed through a flow cuvette positioned in a light beam and the light is scattered by the cells which pass through the beam. The illumination of the cells may be direct (bright field) or indirect (dark field). The illuminated cells are viewed by a photodetector and the number of light flashes are counted. Cell sizes are discriminated by light intensity, and the threshold settings regulate the sensitivity of the photodetector.

One company is currently developing an optical cell counter using a "soft" laser and a unique flow chamber design.

■ **Which parameters are actually measured on the Coulter model S (Sr) and which are calculated by the computer?**

RBC count, WBC count, hemoglobin, and MCV (from summated RBC volume) are actually measured. From these parameters, the remainder are calculated: hematocrit, MCH, and MCHC.

■ **What is the purpose of air segmentation in Technicon's continuous flow principle of automated analysis?**

In continuous flow analysis, all samples are carried through the same analysis pathway and the accuracy of the methodology hinges on minimizing sample interaction—in other words, the previous sample must be adequately washed out to avoid affecting the results of subsequent samples. Without air segmentation, fluid flow through the tubing is streamlined; the layers nearest the tubing wall move more slowly than the fluid in the center. The result of this outer layer hanging back is contamination of the samples which follow. The air segmentation is used to greatly reduce washing time between samples. The surface tension at the air/fluid interface holds the liquid segment together and leaves only a very thin wetting layer on the tubing wall after the segment has passed.

■ **How is protein removed from samples in the autoanalyzer system?**

The autoanalyzer uses dialysis to separate soluble chemical constituents from the proteins in a nondestructive manner. The diluted sample (usually serum) and the recipient reagent stream flow in parallel pathways that are separated by a semipermeable membrane. Proteins, because they are in the size range of colloidal particles, cannot diffuse through the membrane along with the truly dissolved substances and so they are left behind. Dialysis occurs in both directions but is never carried to completion. Preheating of the dialyzing streams and constant temperature control are essential to reproducible dialysis and to the accuracy of the ultimate test result.

■ **Most automated systems other than those of the Technicon company are described as "discrete analysis" systems. What does this mean?**

In discrete systems each sample reaction is handled in a separate compartment and does not come into contact with another sample. The exact physical arrangement of the system has several variations; individual sets of tubes that are washed before the next sample is introduced, or disposable reaction vessels, or even individual packages that contain all the required premeasured reagents. In some cases these packages are used as the cuvette for reading colorimetric reactions.

■ **What is a potentiometric recorder and how does it work?**

A potentiometer is a device used to accurately measure voltage (electrical potential) by a null-balance technique. The unknown voltage is introduced into the potentiometer circuit so that it opposes (in polarity) a known reference voltage. The value of the unknown is measured by comparison to determine the voltage required to exactly oppose the flow of current in the test circuit. This same principle is incorporated in the potentiometric recorder to produce a continuously balancing null-point instrument with a written record. The input signal is compared to the reference signal in a differential amplifier. If the signals are not identical, the difference (error voltage) is amplified sufficiently to drive a servo motor attached to a recording pen and slidewire resistor. Any fraction of the reference voltage may be selected for comparison by moving the sliding contact to the proper point on the slidewire. The servo (*L.* slave) motor simply seeks out the null-balance point on the slidewire by trial and error voltage.

■ **How is the photomultiplier tube used to detect gamma radiation?**

The photomultiplier detects light flashes produced when gamma radiation is absorbed by a scintillator material and emitted as a pulse of visible or UV light. The scintillator may be a crystal attached directly to the photomultiplier envelope or a liquid in which the sample is dispersed.

■ **What is analog information?**

Information which is electronically represented as a varying voltage or current is said to be analog in nature. The signal is an electrical analogy representing the varying input parameter (e.g., light intensity, pressure, temperature). Meters and gauges are examples of analog type readout devices that translate the signals into a physical displacement of the indicator needle.

■ **What is digital information?**

Information represented as discrete integers is referred to as digital information. A digital computer electronically represents data as individual numbers (binary) and actually solves problems by doing simple arithmetic. Digital readout devices on laboratory instruments display the result (e.g., %T or concentration units) as integers and eliminate errors possible in reading meter scales. Analog-to-digital converters are circuits that can convert the former electrical signal into the latter for the readout device or a computer interface.

■ **What is meant by the term "hardware" and "software"?**

Computer hardware refers to the mechanical and electrical components of a computer system. Computer software is the set of codes and instructions (i.e., programs) required to make the computer system operate.

■ **Distinguish between the terms "on-line" and "off-line."**

These terms describe the relationship between a terminal or interfaced laboratory instrument and the computer CPU (central processing unit). If the communication is direct, the relationship is said to be on-line. If the data from the terminal or instrument is collected and temporarily stored (e.g., on punched cards, magnetic tape, or punched paper tape) and must be brought to the computer by the user the relationship is described as off-line. When an instrument is said to be interfaced with the computer, it implies that information is transmitted to the computer (on-line) or temporary data storage (off-line) without human inter-vention.

■ **What is a bit?**

Digital computers perform operations on information coded as discrete integers based on the binary number system. A bit is the smallest piece of information that the computer deals with—the BInary digiT (either 1 or 0).

■ **What is meant by machine language and alphanumeric language?**

Machine language is the binary coded information that the computer actually understands and uses to perform its operations. Alphanumeric language is any language that contains both letters (alphabet) and numerals. Computer programs are more easily understood by the user when represented in the mnemonic short-hand, called assembly language, which is alphanumeric and closer to standard English.

■ **What is a CRT?**

A cathode ray tube (CRT) is a special form of vacuum tube that can visually display electrical information. It is the "picture tube" of the oscilliscope monitor and the computer terminal dis-play. It consists of an electron gun, which projects a beam of electrons onto a phosphor-coated screen (also the tube's anode); and several electrodes to control the focus, intensity, and position of the beam. The beam can be moved across the screen to produce pictures, waveforms, and alphanumeric displays by electrical sig-nals on the horizontal and vertical deflection electrodes.

■ **Describe two systems for clot detection in coagulation instru-ments.**

In principle, any of the changes resulting from clot formation can be used to establish the time of coagulation: changes in vis-cosity or fluidity, optical transparency, or electrical conductivity. Two techniques commonly used at present are electrical conduc-tivity and transparency. The latter method claims the advantage that no foreign material need be in contact with the test plasma to potentially influence coagulation.

■ **What is the principle of osmolality measurement used in most osmometers?**

Any of the four interrelated colligative properties resulting when any substance is dissolved in a solvent could in theory be used to determine the number of particles in solution and thus the molality: (1) depression of the freezing point, (2) elevation of the boiling point, (3) decrease in the vapor pressure, or (4) increase in the osmotic pressure.

Most instruments measure the depression of the freezing point (compared to that of the pure solvent). The instrument consists of a refrigeration unit, a vibrator, a thermistor to measure the temperature, and a constant current source and a wheatstone bridge balancing circuit. In operation, the sample is rapidly cooled below its freezing point without ice formation (supercooling) and freezing of the unstable liquid is initiated (e.g., by mechanical shock from the vibrator). As the supercooled liquid freezes, the formation of crystals liberates heat and the temperature of the sample rises to its true freezing point. The freezing point is measured by the thermistor and balancing circuit during the equilibrium period, which lasts until freezing is complete. Temperature is measured electrically by the balancing circuit as a function of the thermistor resistance.

■ **What two methods can be used to verify the accuracy of an autodilutor?**

The accuracy of both sample aspiration and diluent delivery can be determined gravimetrically using water in weighed vials. Generally an average value of several aspirations or deliveries is determined. If the dilution ratio is the major concern, the results of macrodilutions with volumetric glassware can be compared with those of the dilutor using spectrophotometry. A dye such as ferroin (phenanthroline ferrous sulfate complex), which absorbs at 508 nm and follows Beer's law over a wide range of concentration, is used as the sample to be diluted.

■ **List the basic components of a gas-liquid chromatograph.**

The basic components of a gas-liquid chromatograph are: (1) injection port, (2) column, (3) column oven, including temperature controls, (4) detector, including temperature controls, (5) electrometer or power supply (depending on detector type), and (6) recorder.

■ **List three types of detectors for gas chromatography.**

Three types of detectors for gas chromatography are: (1) thermal conductivity detector, (2) flame ionization detector, and (3) electron capture detector.

■ **What is the basic principle of separations by gas-liquid chromatography (GLC)?**

Any material which is volatile or can be converted into a volatile derivative can be analyzed by GLC. The separation is based on the difference in solubility of the material between the carrier gas phase and the inert liquid phase coated on the column walls or packing. The sample is vaporized at the injection port and is swept into the column by the carrier gas. The sample components partition themselves between the two phases on the basis of their individual diffusion rates and their relative solubilities in the liquid phase. The result is that components move through the column at different rates and appear at different times at the detector. The time of retention in the column is characteristic for the sample component and the analysis conditions and is rarely identical for two compounds. Passage through the detector generates an analog signal that is recorded on a moving chart. The component can be identified by its retention time in comparison with that of an internal standard and quantitated by integration of the peak area. The gas chromatograph can be interfaced with a mass spectrometer to provide the ultimate in sample separation and identification.

■ **Distinguish between the terms "accuracy" and "precision."**

Accuracy describes how closely an experimental result approaches the true value of the quantity being measured. Precision describes the reproducibility of repeated measurements on the same sample and is an indication of the cumulative effect of all random experimental errors inherent in the procedure. It is easily possible for a method to yield precise results and to be entirely inaccurate.

■ **What is the purpose of quality control in the clinical laboratory?**

Quality control programs are designed to assure that laboratory results are reliable, that is, both accurate and precise, on a day-to-day basis.

■ **What is the place of statistical evaluation in the quality control program?**

Since repeated analysis on the same sample (e.g., a control sample) will generally not give identical results, the significance of the cumulative contributions to random error in the method can be adequately evaluated only by statistical methods. A graphical plot of a series of replicate results versus the frequency of occurence of each value would produce a normal bell-shaped (Gaussian) curve with the average value (arithmetic mean) in the center and with approximately half of the values lower and the other half higher than the mean. With a sufficiently large number of aliquots, the mean value will closely approach the true value of the constituent being measured—i.e., to average the result reduces the chance of any one result being erroneous. The precision of the method is indicated by the standard deviation which is a measure of the scatter of values around the mean. The smaller the standard deviation, the greater the precision. Laboratory results are said to be in statistical control when the significant sources of error are known and kept under control as indicated by the results of routine quality control samples, which fall within the prescribed acceptable limits established by statistical evaluation.

■ **Why should a quality control specimen closely resemble the patient samples both chemically and physically?**

The underlying premise is that any patient sample is subject to a series of random experimental errors throughout the course of an analysis. The highest degree of quality control is obtained when control samples are subject to all the same possible errors. Steps in the analysis that may be taken for granted, such as aspiration of the sample in an automated system or protein removal (which an aqueous control would bypass) may remain undisclosed sources of erratic results. The levels and varieties of chemical constituents should be comparable to normal patient values. This will reproduce constant sources of chemical interference as they would be found in an actual patient sample.

■ **What is the significance of a single control value that falls outside the established limits of acceptability?**

Any control sample outside acceptable limits should be evaluated carefully before test results can be reported. Inherent in the statistical design of the quality control limits, which are defined in terms of standard deviation from the mean, is the fact that a known percentage of individual values will fall outside. For example: if the acceptable limits of a procedure are set as the mean ±2 s.d., we can be statistically confident that this interval encloses 95% of the values that would be obtained by repeated analysis of the control sample. The 95% confidence level also assures us that 5%, or 1 out of 20 results, will be outside these limits and not indicate any problem in the analysis conditions. The crux of the matter in evaluating an individual result that falls outside the limits is to determine whether this represents a true problem or is simply the 1 in 20 we should expect. If no analysis problem is obvious, we would approach the dilemma by selecting a new control sample and repeating the analysis on it as well as on several patient samples chosen at random from those which have already been run. If the new control value is now within limits and the patient values are confirmed, we can assume that the procedure is still in control. Even though the control value has been explained, both values should be recorded on the quality control chart. If the new control is still outside the limits, it may indicate a serious problem and the analysis must be scrutinized step by step.

■ **What is the significance of a trend or shift in a quality control chart?**

From the normal frequency distribution curve (bell-shaped curve) of statistics, we should expect daily values to vary from the mean so that on the average half the values are above and half the values are below the mean.

Control values which show a sustained increase or decrease over several days exhibit a trend away from the mean. The trend may indicate deterioration in reagents, instrumentation, or even the control sample pool, and must be investigated.

Control values that appear to distribute themselves on one side of the mean for several days may have taken a shift and should also arouse suspicion and investigation.

■ **Is quality control necessary with automated instrument systems?**

Absolutely! Not only should controls be run daily on such systems, they should be interspersed through each batch of samples. One of the desirable qualities of automation may be the increased speed and precision with which the system can repeat manipulations, but the increased complexity of operations provides more sources of error from miscalibration. An inadequately supervised instrument will continue to produce results as long as you let it, but accuracy to accompany the precision may be entirely accidental.

CHAPTER 8

Chemistry

This chapter is both review and overview. You are reminded to return to your (perhaps dusty) biochemistry textbook and to clinical texts containing specific methodologies for details which you may have forgotten or have not as yet fully appreciated. We hope that this overview will refresh your memory, tie together loose ends, and perhaps provide a perspective to the applications of undergraduate chemistry.

LIPIDS, PROTEINS, AND CARBOHYDRATES

JOAN SHROUT

■ **What are the plasma lipids?**

Plasma lipids include phospholipids, sterols such as cholesterol and cholesterol esters, mono-, di-, and triglycerides, and non-esterified fatty acids. Total lipid analysis also includes fat soluble vitamins.

■ **Give the general functions of plasma lipids in the body.**

In general, lipids are required as components of cellular and subcellular membranes (phospholipid, cholesterol), as a source of energy to tissue, as components for other substances (cholesterol for steroid hormones and vitamins, and phospholipid for thromboplastin), as insulation and padding for organs, and as components for neural myelin sheaths.

■ **Where and how does lipid synthesis occur?**

Most of the endogenous plasma lipids are synthesized by the liver, the overall metabolic pathway having many steps.

The exogenous lipid molecules are ingested and broken down to varying degrees in the intestine by the bile acids and pancreatic secretions (e.g., lipase). Formation of chylomicrons occurs in the intestinal cells and via the lymphatics and systemic circulation they go to adipose tissue where they are either hydrolyzed or resynthesized, or the chylomicrons go to the liver.

In the liver the exogenous molecules are disassembled and then rebuilt (as demonstrated by radioactive tagging). The synthesis of protein also occurs in the liver, and normally the "rebuilt" lipids are conjugated with a specific protein forming the lipoprotein.

Lipids can be acquired exogenously from the diet or can be derived endogenously. The latter is especially true of cholesterol, which can be synthesized from acetate groups in most organ tissues.

■ **What are lipoproteins and how are they classified?**

Lipoproteins are lipid-protein complexes (about 30% protein) which function in the transport of lipids.

Electrophoretically the lipoprotein mobilities match those of the globulins, leading to classification as alpha, pre-beta, and beta. Chylomicrons are also detected by electrophoresis, as a nonmigrating band at the point of origin, although serum from a fasting patient should normally reveal no chylomicron band. Normally the alpha is the principal carrier of phospholipid (30%); the pre-beta carries mainly triglyceride (44%) and some cholesterol (18%); the beta is the chief carrier of cholesterol (43%), as well as albumin, which transports the fatty acids.

By ultracentrifugation the lipoproteins are separated into very light density lipoprotein, VLDL (pre-beta), light density lipoprotein, LDL (beta), and high density lipoprotein, HDL (alpha).

■ **What are sources of error encountered in lipid profile testing?**

Lipid testing must be performed after a 12- to 14-hour fast. The patient should be on a normal diet 7 days prior to testing. Lipoprotein studies should not be performed for 6 weeks after myocardial infarct. Care should be taken to prevent bacterial contamination of blood specimen, as this may lead to unclear electrophoretic pattern as well as possible increase of triglyceride and increased anodic migration of beta and pre-beta bands. (Add 1.5% thimerosal to serum to prevent bacterial growth.) Specimens should not be frozen, as this also may lead to loss of clear bands. Lipid abnormalities can be of two classes: hypolipidemia, a decrease in one or more lipoprotein or lipid (e.g. abetalipoproteinemia, Tangiers disease), or hyperlipidemia, an increase in one or more lipoprotein or lipid.

■ **What is lipid phenotyping?**

Table 7. Predominant characteristics found in each of the five types of hyperlipidemia (classification of Fredrickson, Levy, and Lees)

	Description	Lipid pattern	Serum	Other
Type I	Familial fat-induced hyperlipidemia Rare	Chylomicrons present Triglycerides increased Cholesterol increased (usually)	Turbid; creamy supernatant with clear infranate	Deficiency of lipoproteinlipase Alpha and beta fractions reduced, no pre-beta
Type IIA	Familial hyper-beta lipoproteinemia Common	Increased beta band; cholesterol markedly elevated Normal pre-beta	Clear	
Type IIB	Familial hyper-beta lipoproteinemia Common	Increased beta band; cholesterol markedly elevated Increased pre-beta band; slight moderate elevation of triglyceride; LDL ratio >190 mg/dl	Slightly turbid without chylomicron layer	
Type III	Familial hyper-beta and pre-beta lipoproteinemia Uncommon, but not rare	Abnormal beta (light density, <1.006 g/ml) with high amount of cholesterol Increase in Sf 12-20 and Sf 20-100 Cholesterol and triglyceride elevated, cholesterol > triglyceride	Turbid	Abnormal glucose tolerance Only genetic causes*
Type IV	Carbohydrate-induced hyperlipemia Common	Distinct pre-beta band; elevated triglyceride Normal or slightly elevated cholesterol; LDL ratio <190 mg/dl	Turbid or clear	Abnormal glucose tolerance Obesity
Type V	Familial hyperchylomicronemia Rare	High levels of chylomicrons and pre-beta Cholesterol increased Triglycerides increased	Turbid; creamy supernatant with lipemic infranate	Abnormal glucose tolerance

*The other types listed can occur secondary to other disorders, (e.g., liver disease, pancreatitis), which must be carefully considered in regard to treatment of the lipidemia.

Phenotyping is the classification of hyperlipidemias into five main types. The classification is based upon ultracentrifugation results, or the electrophoretic pattern of serum, in agreement with specific lipid fraction tests, especially cholesterol and triglyceride. Each of the five types has a characteristic pattern of specific lipid and lipoprotein elevation (see Table 7).

■ **What are the major plasma proteins?**

Identified by electrophoretic separation on cellulose acetate, the plasma proteins are albumin, alpha-1-globulins, alpha-2-globulins, beta globulins, and gamma globulins.

■ **What are the general functions of plasma proteins in the body?**

Ingested proteins can be broken down into amino acids and subsequently resynthesized into required body proteins. Amino acids are utilized to build muscle tissue and to synthesize enzymes and hormones. Proteins are the principal transport system in the body. Water insoluble lipids, drugs, hormones, and many cations are carried by specific proteins. Proteins, especially albumin, contribute to maintenance of normal osmotic pressure and water distribution.

■ **Where is the site of protein synthesis?**

The plasma proteins are synthesized in the liver, with the exception of the gamma globulins and some beta globulins. Because of this, the albumin/globulin (A/G) ratio and tests based on it—ceph floccs, thymol turbidity—were performed to detect liver damage. The gamma globulins are synthesized and transported by lymphocytes (B-cells) and plasma cells. Some beta globulins are made elsewhere in the RE system.

The liver is also the major site for breakdown of protein. Some amino acids return to the "amino acid pool." Others undergo breakdown: through a series of reactions ammonia is formed, which is converted to urea nitrogen (in the liver). The blood urea nitrogen (BUN) is normally cleared by the kidney.

■ **Discuss the purpose of the oral glucose tolerance test, and the characteristic insulin response patterns of diabetes, hypoglycemia, and the "normal" individual.**

The glucose tolerance will test the rate of removal of a specific carbohydrate—glucose—from the bloodstream. The rate at which glucose is absorbed in the gastrointestinal tract, as well as the rate and degree of filtration and reabsorption by the kidney, are factors that may influence the tolerance curve. Malabsorption syndrome (in the intestine) can occur, resulting in a "flat" curve. Low or normal plasma glucose levels with glucose in the urine may indicate a condition called renal glycosuria.

In the normal individual the insulin response to an oral glucose load is almost immediate, with the insulin level peaking between 30 and 60 minutes. This results in the plasma glucose level peaking between 30 and 60 minutes and returning to normal limits within 3 hours.

In "maturity onset" diabetes the secretion of insulin is delayed, followed by a slightly higher than normal level at 2 hours. The blood glucose is therefore usually elevated until around the 2-hour point. In overt diabetes there is little or no secretion of insulin, resulting in abnormally elevated glucose levels throughout the testing.

Hypoglycemia is characterized by delayed secretion of insulin, followed by hypersecretion, which is believed to be the effect of prolonged stimulation to the pancreas by the elevated glucose. The blood glucose is usually below normal after the 2-hour point, through 4 and 5 hours, because of the high insulin levels.

There are various criteria to evaluate tolerance results. One commonly used is a point system (Wilkerson) with the fasting and 3-hour specimen results worth 1 point each if the result (glucose in mg/dl) is above normal limits, and the 1-hour and 2-hour results each worth ½ point if abnormally high. A score of 2 or greater indicates diabetes mellitus.

■ **What are sources of error in glucose tolerance testing?**

Incorrect preparation of the patient can lead to erroneous results. The patient must be fasting and must be given a glucose load calculated for his body mass. Also, the patient must have eaten adequate carbohydrates (150 gm/day) for 72 hours prior to testing. The patient should not have been subjected to recent trauma (surgery, myocardial infarct, labor and delivery, and so on).

■ **Which hormones contribute to the regulation of the blood glucose level?**

Two hormones directly regulate the blood glucose. Glucagon and insulin are both produced in the pancreas, in the alpha and beta cells of the islet of Langerhans, respectively. The secretion of glucagon accelerates the breakdown of glycogen (glycogenolysis) in the liver, causing a rise in blood glucose. Secretion of insulin results in an increased permeability of certain cellular membranes to glucose. It further stimulates formation of glycogen from glucose in the liver, thereby reducing blood glucose levels.

Other hormones also contribute to glucose metabolism. ACTH and growth hormone from the pituitary, 11-oxy-21 steroids from the adrenal cortex, epinephrine from the adrenal medulla, and thyroxine from the thyroid exert effects in the metabolic pathways of glucose.

■ **List other carbohydrate tolerance tests.**

Tolerance tests can also be performed for pentoses, lactose, galactose, and D-xylose.

■ **What is the purpose of a tolbutamide tolerance?**

Tolbutamide (Orinase) is a hypoglycemic agent that acts by stimulating the pancreatic beta cells to produce insulin. Delayed or low production of insulin occurs in some adult individuals and is termed "maturity onset" diabetes. The glucose levels after tolbutamide stimulation have distinctive patterns compared to nondiabetic response to tolbutamide. Abnormal response to this tolerance can also indicate adenoma of the pancreas.

■ **What is the significance of lactic acid?**

Lactic acid is a metabolite of anaerobic glucose metabolism

Table 8. Reference methods as well as one or two of the commonly performed procedures for tests discussed in this chapter

Test	Reference method	Routine clinical method
Total lipid	Sperry and Brand; gravimetric	Phosphovanillin
Cholesterol	Abell; gravimetric	Lieberman-Burchard
Triglyceride	Van Handel; gravimetric; glycerol determination, with phospholipid removed by zeolite	Glycerol determination with Hantzsche (acetylacetone) color reaction Enzymatic
Total protein	Kjeldahl; gravimetric; determination of protein nitrogen	Biuret
Glucose	Hexokinase; enzymatic; glucose oxidase, enzymatic (although inhibitors may be present)	Alkaline ferricyanide; cupric neocuprine
Calcium	Clark-Collip; titration of calcium oxalate with potassium permanganate or ceric ion	8-OH-quinoline Atomic absorption
Chloride	Schales and Schales; titration with mercuric nitrate	Cotlove chloridometers
Carbon dioxide	Van Slyke; gasometric	

within the muscle tissue (tricarboxylic acid cycle). Strenuous exercise or muscle trauma will result in elevated lactate levels. Normally, this is removed (detoxified) by the liver. In liver dysfunction, however, the blood lactate level rises. Decreased cardiac output (e.g., congestive heart failure) may also contribute to rising lactate levels because of decreased oxygen delivery to the tissues.

• • •

Table 8 lists the reference methods for some test analyses commonly performed in clinical chemistry. The exact methodology and procedure can be found in textbooks. It is of some importance to be acquainted with the reference method in terms of understanding inherent error, e.g., measurement of glucose on the autoanalyzer versus "true glucose" values. While this descrepancy does not produce problems routinely in the clinical laboratory, the technologist should be aware that such a discrepancy or variance among methodologies does exist and should have some concept of the underlying reasons for the variance.

HORMONES AND ENZYMES

ANTHONY CAFARO

■ **What is an enzyme?**

An enzyme is a protein product of living cells which catalyzes chemical reactions independent of the cell.

■ **How is the synthesis of enzymes controlled?**

Enzymes are under genetic control—one gene, one polypeptide.

■ **What is their composition?**

Enzymes are composed of two principal components. The apoenzyme portion is protein, thermolabile, and nondialyzable, and the coenzyme portion is organic, thermostable, and dialyzable.

■ **Are enzymes always immediately active upon their formation?**

No. Many enzymes exist in an inactive form, referred to as a preenzyme or proemzyme. These substances sometimes require the presence of activators which may be ionic or nonionic. Such substances are: magnesium, cobalt, manganese, hormones, catecholamines, and other enzymes.

■ **Can enzymatic action be inactivated?**

Yes. Enzymes may be inactivated both in vivo and in vitro. Substances such as cyanide, mercury, arsenicals, carbon monoxide, and certain narcotics are sulfhydryl inhibitors. In vitro inactivation is related to the protein nature of the enzyme and is principally concerned with changes in temperature and pH.

■ **Where are enzymes located within the cell?**

Enzymes may be located within the cytoplasm of the cell, within the subcellular organelles, or within the nucleus. The cytoplasmic enzymes are the more primitive and principally carry on anaerobic metabolism. This includes some of the transaminases, peptidases, and phosphorylases, as well as enzymes required for fatty acid synthesis and glycolysis. When cellular damage occurs, these enzymes are the first to appear in the serum. Lysosomes contain acid phosphatase, ribonuclease, and cathepsin. Incomplete phagocytosis occurs when these enzymes are deficient. Within the mitochondria are enzymes principally concerned with aerobic metabolism that are most affected by poison such as cyanide, which destroys the oxidative capacity of the cell. When these enzymes appear elevated in the serum, they are indicative of a more advanced degree of cellular destruction. Microsomes contain alkaline phosphatase, esterases, and enzymes for both lipid and protein synthesis. The nucleus contains enzymes for glycolysis and nucleic acid synthesis.

■ **What is the clinical significance of enzymatic localization?**

Inasmuch as similar enzymes are located in different portions of the cell, the appearance of the specific isoenzymes within the serum may denote the degree of cellular damage. For example, the glutamic oxalacetic transaminase is located both in the cytoplasm and within the mitochondria of the cell. The appearance of the mitochondrial fraction denotes more extensive cellular damage.

■ **How are enzymes named?**

Enzymes are named on the basis of the substrate upon which they react, followed by a suffix which denotes the type of action the enzyme exerts upon the substrate; for example, lactic acid dehydrogenase—the substrate is lactic acid, the function is to remove hydrogen.

■ **What is the definition of a standard unit?**

One standard unit is the amount of enzyme that catalyzes the conversion of one micromole (microequivalent) of substrate or coenzyme per minute under defined conditions of the test (the usual recommended temperature is 25° C). The pH is variable and must be adjusted for the optimum reactivity of the particular enzyme.

■ **What are the factors which affect enzyme activity?**

Temperature, pH, substrate concentration, and enzyme concentration all affect enzyme activity.

■ **What is the effect of temperature upon an enzymatic reaction?**

The activity of most enzymes increases by a factor of 1.4 to 2 for each 10° C increment between 10 and 30° C. A temperature difference of 1° C may affect the activity by 4 to 10%.

■ **What relationship should reaction rate bear to substrate concentration in enzyme determinations?**

When testing for enzymes, the rate of the reaction should not be affected by substrate concentration; that is, the addition of more substrate will not alter the rate of enzymatic activity. This is referred to as zero order kinetics.

■ **What is meant by first order kinetics in enzyme determinations?**

First order kinetics in enzyme determinations relates to the activity of the enzyme being proportional to its concentration; that is, the more enzyme present, the faster the reactions. All enzyme reactions should be first order kinetics with respect to enzyme concentration and zero order with respect to substrate concentration.

■ **What is the general classification of enzymes?**

A general classification of clinical enzymes includes oxidases, dehydrogenases, transferases, hydrolases, lyases, and isomerases.

■ **What is an isoenzyme?**

Isoenzymes are enzymes that react on a similar substrate but may differ in their chemical properties, that is, pH optima and relative charge.

■ **What is the character of the lactic acid dehydrogenase isoenzymes and how are they designated?**

By electrophoresis, five distinct bands are identified. The most cathodic, LDH fraction 5, migrates with the gammaglobulins. All the other fractions migrate toward the anode. Some confusion exists regarding the nomenclature inasmuch as some have reversed the order. However, dominantly in the literature the most anodic fraction is fraction 1, which is the heart fraction; fraction 5, the liver fraction, is the slowest. In this discussion this is the format that will be followed.

■ **How may one make an assessment of these enzymes without having the capability of electrophoresis?**

This may be accomplished by measuring the total lactic acid

dehydrogenase activity followed by determination of the heat-resistant fraction of LDH; fraction 1 resists denaturation at 58° C for 30 minutes, while the activity of the other four isoenzymes is destroyed under these conditions. This may also be confirmed by the performance of an alpha-hydroxy butyric dehydrogenase determination directly. The activity of this enzyme parallels that of the LDH fraction 1.

■ **Are the lactic acid dehydrogenase and isoenzyme determinations valid after freezing serum?**

No. Fractions 4 and 5 are rapidly destroyed by freezing and are diminished on storage at 4° C. Some investigators have noted that no significant alteration occurs in the activity of the isoenzymes if the sera are stored at room temperature up to 10 days.

■ **Can isoenzyme determinations of LDH be determined by alternate methods?**

Yes. Biochemical inhibition methods utilizing oxalate are used to inhibit the fast isoenzymes and urea to inhibit the isoenzymes of low electrophoretic mobility. Others have noted that pyruvate enhances the activity of the LDH fraction 1 in the presence of urea and thus have used the LDH isoenzyme index utilizing 2 molar lactate and .02 molar lactate plus 2 molar urea as substrate.

■ **Is there ever a clinical situation in which more than 5 lactic acid dehydrogenase isoenzyme bands may be seen?**

Yes. If an isoenzyme determination is done on seminal fluid, an X-band will appear having a mobility lying between LDH fractions 3 and 4. This band is characteristic of the mature testes and is observed in seminal plasma in relation to the number of spermatozoa present; that is, if the patient is aspermic, the LDH fraction X will not be present.

■ **What enzymes are clinically useful in the evaluation of myocardial disease, principally infarction?**

The enzymes that are principally concerned with evaluation of myocardial damage are lactic acid dehydrogenase, serum glutamic oxalacetic transaminase, creatinine phosphokinase, and alpha-hydroxy butyric dehydrogenase.

■ **Is any one of the above tests totally specific for myocardial damage?**

No. All of the enzymes mentioned above may be elevated in both striated muscle disease and some liver diseases.

■ **How then can one make a more useful evaluation of myocardial damage using the same enzymes?**

A more useful evaluation can be made by the performance of isoenzyme determinations of both lactic acid dehydrogenase and creatinine phosphokinase. This separation of enzymes may be accomplished by electrophoresis wherein the most anodic fractions of lactic acid dehydrogenase, fraction 1 and 2, are associated with myocardial damage. Both the intermediate and third fractions of CPK are associated with myocardial damage.

■ **Are isoenzyme determinations helpful if the clinical history is compatible with myocardial infarction but the lactic acid dehydrogenase determination and the CPK determination are normal?**

Yes. Diagnostic shifts in the isoenzyme fractionation have been noted before the clinical manifestation of abnormal elevation of either of the above-mentioned enzymes is present. Therefore, when the clinical situation dictates, isoenzyme determinations may be helpful.

■ **Can one expect any single "cardiac enzyme" to be elevated earlier than the others when suspected myocardial damage is present?**

Although at various times authors have reported that the creatinine phosphokinase activity is the earliest to be seen, there is no hard and fast rule. Generally, in the decreasing order of clinical specificity, the cardiac enzymes are related to each other thus: lactic acid dehydrogenase with isoenzyme determination and creatinine phosphokinase with isoenzyme determination and hydroxy butyric dehydrogenase. It must be remembered that LDH isoenzymes and CPK isoenzymes may be altered prior to the appearance of elevated total activity.

■ **Where is creatine phosphokinase located?**

Creatine phosphokinase is located in skeletal muscle, striated muscle, and brain.

■ **How many isoenzyme bands are there for creatine phosphokinase?**

Three—a fast band associated with brain tissue, an intermediate band which is associated with heart tissue, and a slow band which is associated with heart and with skeletal muscle.

■ **Which enzymes are clinically useful in evaluating hepatic disease?**

Serum glutamic oxalacetic transaminase, serum glutamic pyruvic transaminase, lactic acid dehydrogenase with isoenzyme determination, and isocitrate dehydrogenase aid in evaluating hepatic disease. When jaundice is present and the differential diagnosis of intrahepatic and extrahepatic jaundice is at issue, gammaglutamyl transpeptidase and adenosine deaminase are of increased importance.

■ **Which enzymes are the most widely used in the clinical laboratory for the diagnosis of hepatic disease?**

The two transaminases, SGOT and SGPT, are the most widely used.

■ **In what situations may the greatest magnitude of rise be demonstrated in the elevation of these enzymes?**

In acute hepatitis and acute toxic injury to the liver, serum activity may be elevated 20 to 30 times normal.

■ **Of what use is the SGOT/SGPT ratio?**

The normal ratio is 1:1. A reversed ratio is almost always seen in acute hepatitis. In chronic hepatitis and cirrhosis, a ratio greater than 1:1 is usually noted.

■ **How many isoenzyme bands are produced on electrophoresis of the glutamic oxalacetic transaminase?**

Two bands are demonstrated. A fast band, which is distributed in the cytoplasm located principally in heart and liver tissue, and a slow band located in the mitochondria, seen in massive liver necrosis.

■ **Of what value is lactic acid dehydrogenase determination in liver disease?**

Total activity in the serum is nonspecific; however, fractionation of LDH into isoenzymes is valuable in that the elevation of the fraction 5 band is a sensitive indicator for parenchymal damage. Increases may be seen in acute parenchymal necrosis, space-occupying lesions, and congestive failure. It must be remembered, however, that fraction 5 elevations may also be seen with striated muscle injury. However, history and SGPT determinations are helpful in making the differential.

■ **Can drugs have an effect upon the activity of serum glutamic oxalacetic transaminase and lactic acid dehydrogenase?**

Yes. Opiates may cause a secondary rise in serum glutamic oxalacetic transaminase and lactic acid dehydrogenase by their effect on the hepatic cell. The performance of lactic acid dehydrogenase isoenzyme determinations will demonstrate this effect by an elevation of the LDH fraction 5 (cathodic fraction). Also, pregnancy and oral contraceptives may cause an elevation of both SGOT and LDH.

■ **What drugs may induce liver disease?**

Two categories of drugs injurious to the liver are recognized: (1) predicable and dose-related drugs such as the protoplasmic poisons (e.g., carbon tetrachloride and inorganic phosphorus); (2) drugs that act in a somewhat more unpredictable manner, affecting cell metabolism or via an idiosyncrasy of the host. Antibiotics such as tetracycline and antimetabolites such as mercaptopurine are examples of the former. Chlorpromazine is an example of the latter. Intermediate is methyl testosterone, which is toxic and also causes jaundice (cholestatic). Certain of the oral contraceptives containing testosterone derivatives can have a similar effect.

■ **Can enzymes be used to detect hepatitis when jaundice does not exist?**

Yes. Transaminases may be elevated as early as 1 to 4 weeks prior to the clinical onset of jaundice in a patient with hepatitis. Additionally, lactic acid dehydrogenase isoenzyme determinations may demonstrate a prominent fraction 5 prior to the appearance of clinical disease.

■ **Can drugs be a cause of spurious elevations in the serum glutamic oxalacetic transaminase?**

Yes. It has been shown that PAS (para-aminosalicylic acid), a drug commonly used in the treatment of tuberculosis, can interfere with the colorimetric reaction that is sometimes used to determine the serum glutamic oxalacetic transaminase activity. Most of these problems can be circumvented by using a reaction that requires a coenzyme such as nicotinamide adenine dinucleotide (NAD) as an intermediary reaction. The absorbance of NAD occurs in the ultraviolet range and thereby will circumvent any interfering color-producing reactions.

■ **Which of the common enzymes are affected by hemolysis?**

When hemolysis is present, lactic acid dehydrogenase and aldolase determinations may be significantly elevated. Lesser elevations in the order of decreasing amounts are gammaglutamyl transpeptidase, serum glutamic oxalacetic transaminase, isocitrate dehydrogenase, leucine aminopeptidase, and glutamic pyruvic transaminase.

■ **Which enzymes are most often elevated in biliary tract disease associated with cholestasis?**

The three enzymes most often measured associated with clinical biliary tract disease are nonspecific alkaline phosphatase, leucine aminopeptidase, and 5' nucleotidase.

■ **What additional information may be obtained from the determination of alkaline phosphatase isoenzyme?**

If one performs an alkaline phosphatase isoenzyme determination, a significant liver band is noted. This usually migrates in polyacrylamide gel in the area of the alpha-2 globulin. The beta-1 position is occupied by alkaline phosphatase of bone or placental origin, and the fraction which migrates in the beta-2 area is associated with the intestinal alkaline phosphatase.

■ **What other enzymes are clinically useful in biliary tract disease?**

Gammaglutamyl transpeptidase may be significantly altered in cases of obstructive jaundice.

■ **Where is gammaglutamyl transpeptidase located and what is its clinical significance?**

Gammaglutamyl transpeptidase is located in liver, pancreas, and kidney tissue. Its principal value is in determining the cause of jaundice. In cases of hepatocellular and obstructive jaundice the gammaglutamyl transpeptidase tends to be disproportionately more elevated than the transaminase. The reverse is true in viral hepatitis.

■ **Why do biliary tract enzymes become elevated in cases of infectious or toxic hepatitis?**

In clinical cases of hepatitis, the elevation of the biliary enzymes is a result of the cholestatic phase of the illness, which may be seen in both acute and chronic situations.

■ **What are some other causes for elevation of the biliary tract enzymes?**

All three enzymes, that is, nonspecific alkaline phosphatase, 5' nucleotidase, and leucine aminopeptidase, may be elevated in association with drug therapy.

■ **Which drugs are most commonly associated with cholestatic jaundice?**

Sulfonylurea derivatives: namely, phenothiazine tranquilizers such as chlorpromazine, sulfonamides, antidiabetic drugs, and oral diuretics; anabolic steroids such as androgens and certain of the antibiotics, principally erythromycin estolate; are associated with cholestatic jaundice.

■ **Can oral contraceptives (the Pill) be associated with jaundice?**

Yes. Most instances of jaundice associated with the Pill are seen during the first three cycles of its administration. If jaundice occurs after this time, it is felt that it most likely is not related to the Pill. For this reason it is felt that prescreening for hepatic disease be performed prior to a patient being given the Pill. Other interferences caused by the drug include alteration in glucose metabolism and alterations in T4 and T3 results.

■ **What enzymes are useful in the determination of muscle disease not of cardiac origin?**

Creatine phosphokinase, aldolase, and lactic acid dehydrogenase, particularly with isoenzyme determination, are useful determinants.

■ **Can spurious elevations of these enzymes be seen?**

Yes. Elevations of these enzymes may be noted following strenuous exercise. Sometimes the peak is observed between 16 and 24 hours and may remain elevated for as long as 48 hours. Physical conditioning of the subject may alter the response of these enzymes.

■ **In what clinical situations may these muscle enzymes be altered?**

The most striking increases in the muscle enzymes occur in progressive Duchenne type of muscular dystrophy. It has been also noted that elevations may be seen in siblings of affected children. Muscular dystrophy usually affects males, and children at age 6 months have been shown to have elevated values of these enzymes only to be followed by the appearance of clinical signs and symptoms at some time later. Other types of dystrophies usually are associated with elevated values but are not as high as those observed in the Duchenne type.

■ **Does inflammation of the muscle cause an alteration of the muscle enzymes?**

Serum enzyme activity may be seen associated with polymyositis syndrome; these elevations tend to parallel the severity of the disease process.

■ Do the isoenzymes of lactic acid dehydrogenase in any way reflect the type of metabolism carried on in the tissue?

Yes. Fraction 1 is generally associated with aerobic metabolism and is the type observed in cardiac muscle, whereas fraction 5 is associated with anaerobic type of metabolism and is associated with liver and muscle.

■ Under what clinical situations might a very high creatine phosphokinase be seen not associated with significant elevations of aldolase or lactic acid dehydrogenase?

When a cerebral vascular accident (stroke) or malignant hyperthermia are present very high CPK values may be noted.

■ In what situation may a very high lactic acid dehydrogenase be observed without significant elevations of either aldolase or creatine phosphokinase?

This situation is usually seen in cases of hemolytic disease, particularly vitamin B_{12} deficiency (pernicious anemia). In this situation, the serum glutamic oxalacetic transaminases are also normal, and on isoenzyme determination of lactic acid dehydrogenase a very prominent fraction 1 is present.

■ Can malignancy affect enzymes?

Yes. Malignancies, because of multiple system involvement, may cause irregular elevations of all the enzymes. In these situations, there may be no characteristic pattern present unless one system is more severely affected than the others.

■ Is there a clinical value in performing enzyme determinations on body fluids other than plasma?

In cases of malignancy, it is well to perform enzyme determinations on the body fluid in question, particularly lactic acid dehydrogenase with isoenzyme determination; however, in these situations a concurrent serum determination should be performed although these determinations in and of themselves are significant only if there is a notable difference between the body fluid level and that noted in the serum, i.e., body fluid value is higher than serum. Although no direct etiology can be determined in such a situation, it does tend to support the theory that active tissue damage is occurring in the area and producing a change in the body fluid. (Body fluids refer to cerebral spinal fluid, pleural and abdominal effusions, urine, and articular fluid.)

■ If one cannot perform an alkaline phosphatase isoenzyme determination by electrophoresis, is there any other method of determining alkaline phosphatase source?

Yes. Alkaline phosphatase of bone can be distinguished from the hepatic isoenzyme by the fact that bone alkaline phosphatase is more rapidly inactivated at 55° C than that of liver. Approximately one-half of the bone alkaline phosphatase activity can be destroyed within 8 minutes, while the latter requires an incubation of approximately 20 minutes before half of its activity is lowered.

■ **In what clinical situation might one see an elevated alkaline phosphatase with no associated disease?**

In prepuberal children alkaline phosphatases are uniformly elevated during the period of active bone growth, and elevations of total nonspecific alkaline phosphatase may be seen. When a determination of isoenzymes is performed, it is found that liver and bone fractions both may be observed. In pregnancy, progressive elevation of alkaline phosphatase is noted beginning at 15 weeks gestation and progressing to term. Normal values are obtained between the third and sixth postpartum week.

■ **Are significant elevations of alkaline phosphatase in adults ever normal?**

Excluding pregnancy, significant elevations of alkaline phosphatase in an adult must be considered to be associated with disease until proven otherwise.

■ **Are isolated elevations of alkaline phosphatase observed in infants always normal?**

No. Infants with intrahepatic biliary atresia (incomplete formation of the biliary system within the liver) may have marked elevations of alkaline phosphatase activity.

■ **In what situations clinically might a low serum alkaline phosphatase activity be noted unassociated with other enzyme changes?**

An inborn error of metabolism referred to as hypophosphatasia may be associated with low serum alkaline phophatase activity. The cardinal features of this syndrome are an impaired mineralization of bone, associated with reduced tissue and serum alkaline phosphatase activity, accompanied by the presence of phosphoethanolamine in the urine. This type of change may be seen in infants, in children, and in adults. In the latter there is usually a history of pathologic fractures and a childhood history of vitamin D resistant rickets.

■ **In what clinical situations are the highest alkaline phosphatase observed in adults?**

The alkaline phosphatase is very high in Paget's disease, and on electrophoresis a prominent bone band is noted. Additionally, tumors of the bone (osteogenic sarcoma) are associated with high phosphatase activity.

■ **What precautions should be taken when doing alkaline phosphatase determinations?**

Serum is the preferred specimen for alkaline phosphatase activity. Plasma is to be avoided because of the inhibitory effects of the anticoagulants.

■ **Are acid phosphatases as stable as alkaline phosphatase?**

Serum alkaline phosphatase is generally stable at both room temperature and at 4° C; however, acid phosphatase is very unstable.

■ **Of what value is the determination of the immune precipitable alkaline phosphatase?**

It has been shown that a specific antibody directed against placental alkaline phosphatase can be used in immune precipitable techniques and in such a situation elevations of this enzyme may be detected in significant amounts in some cases of malignancy. This enzyme is referred to by some as Regan enzyme.

■ **What may be the reason of some false elevations of alkaline phosphatase?**

If the patient has received albumin derived from the human placenta, a marked elevation in alkaline phosphatase may be noted.

■ **What is the character of the alkaline phosphatase isoenzymes?**

The liver isoenzyme is moderately heat labile, that of bone is extremely heat labile, and that of placental origin is heat stable. Additionally, the enzyme of placental origin is also inhibited by phenylalanine.

■ **Are there any discrepancies in performing acid phosphatase determinations on serum or plasma?**

Yes. Activity of acid phosphatase in serum is generally greater than that observed in plasma. This is probably caused by the liberation of the enzyme from platelets during the process of coagulation.

■ **Is there normally a prostatic fraction present in serum?**

Generally prostatic acid phosphatase is not normally detectable in serum.

■ **What is characteristic of acid phosphatase arising from carcinoma of the prostate?**

The acid phosphatase arising from carcinoma of the prostate is formaldehyde stable, tartrate labile, resistant to copper, and can be inhibited by heparin. Additionally, 40% alcohol can inhibit the prostatic acid phosphatase. Some authors have recommended using alpha-naphthol phosphate as a substrate for acid phosphatase determination when the prostatic fraction is desired because it is thought that alpha-naphthol phosphate is the most specific of all of the common substrates for prostatic acid phosphatase. It is also well to be familiar with the type of substrate that one is using when performing an acid phosphatase determination and also to avoid the use of oxalate, heparin, and fluoride in tubes when drawing blood samples for acid phosphatase determination.

■ **What other clinical situations might cause an elevation of acid phosphatase?**

Operative trauma, vigorous prostate massage, and infarcts (local tissue death) of the prostate are known to cause transient elevations. Gaucher's disease is associated with: striking increases in plasma acid phosphatase activity; disorders of platelets particularly where destruction is excessive; liver disease particularly in cirrhosis; metastatic carcinoma of the liver; obstructive jaundice and hepatitis; bone disease particularly in advanced Paget's and in cases of metastatic carcinoma; certain kidney diseases; hemolytic disease because of the richness of acid phosphatase in the red blood cells; and certain chromosomal abnormalities. In some instances, these elevations can be best evaluated by performing the tests with and without inhibitors.

■ **Which enzymes are useful in the evaluation of pancreatic disease?**

Amylase and lipase are the most useful.

■ **Are there any isoenzymes associated with amylase?**

Yes. Three bands have been observed on separation of serum, presumably arising from pancreatic, salivary, and liver origin. Some believe that the liver supplies most of the amylase which is normally seen in the sera; however, in clinical situations of acute pancreatitis, total amylase elevation in both serum and urine remains one of the single most important aids in confirming a diagnosis. Isoenzymes are less important.

■ **Is the diagnosis of pancreatitis usually based solely on the presence of observed enzyme activity?**

No. Frequently repeated determinations are required before a significant elevation is seen. Helpful in association with these determinations is serum calcium, which if low is supportive evidence of disease. It has been noted in critically ill patients with elevated amylases that if serum calciums are not reduced but rather are normal or elevated, a possibility of hyperparathyroidism should be entertained.

■ **Are there any other factors involved in evaluating amylase elevations?**

Yes. In the presence of renal disease, incomplete clearing of the serum amylase by the kidneys may preclude the efficiency of the test.

■ **What is the significance of elevated serum amylase in patients presenting with acute abdominal pain?**

Elevations of serum amylase can be considered to be indicative of pancreatic disease. In one-third of the cases, this may be accompanied by hypoglycemia. In general, amylase activity is inversely related to the severity of the pancreatic disease. Some authors believe that amylase values over 1,000 Somogyi units are consistent with surgically correctable lesions frequently involving the biliary tract. Amylase activity between 200 and 500 units is associated with a majority of the patients with idiopathic pancreatitis and hemorrhagic pancreatitis.

■ **How soon can one expect an elevation in amylase activity following abdominal pain?**

Within 2 to 12 hours of the onset of acute disease of the pancreas one may expect an elevation of amylase activity, which will return to normal in healing patients by the fourth day.

■ **What other tests can be easily done in an effort to establish a differential diagnosis of acute abdominal pain?**

This somewhat depends on the relative age and sex of the patient. In a young female of childbearing age, in addition to an amylase a slide pregnancy test and screening test for porphobilinogen are logical tests. This again depends on the clinical situation and could be coupled with total LDH, isoenzyme determination, and CPK, the latter two being helpful if cardiac and/or liver disease are responsible for the clinical symptoms. These four tests do not exhaust the diagnostic possibilities as far as abdominal pain is concerned but generally are helpful.

■ **Are urinary amylases important?**

Urine amylase activity is considered by some to be preferential in suspected pancreatic disease principally because urine amylase is more frequently elevated, persists for a longer period of time, and reaches levels higher than that noted in the serum.

■ **Can amylase activity be elevated in nonpancreatic disease?**

The most common causes of nonpancreatic amylase elevation are obstruction to the common biliary duct, peptic ulcer, ovarian disease, and salivary gland disease (mumps).

■ **What are some of the artifacts that may influence amylase activity?**

Opiates, hemolysis, storage of the serum sample at room temperature, and performing the amylase determination within the immediate postoperative period may cause spurious elevations of amylase.

■ **What method is felt to be the best for true amylase activity?**

The saccharogenic method is best because this is the only method which truly demonstrates human isoamylase activity. By this technique, at least three different isoamylases have been noted emanating from the pancreas, salivary gland, and liver. All three have an electrophoretic mobility similar to that of gammaglobulin. The albumin activity is demonstrable only by amyloclastic technique, which is believed to be an artifact.

■ **How may a diagnosis of pancreatitis be ruled out by amylase activity?**

If the amylase level is not increased within the first 24 hours after the onset of symptoms, it is likely that the patient does not have acute pancreatitis.

■ **What other body fluids may be used to make a diagnosis of acute pancreatitis?**

Determination of amylase activity in peritoneal fluid has been found to be an advantage in the diagnosis of acute pancreatitis. Elevations of amylase in the fluid are highly suggestive. Other conditions that may also be associated with elevation of peritoneal fluid amylase are perforated small bowel and ectopic pregnancy.

■ **What is macroamylase?**

In macroamylasemia, the amylase is bound to an immune globulin, either IgA or IgG. This condition has been noted in association with malabsorption secondary to malignant lymphoma and villous atrophy. The reason for the elevated amylase activity is because this large molecule is not readily eliminated by the kidney as is the normal amylase, and because of this nonclearance by the kidney concomitant elevations of amylase are not noted in the urine.

■ **Of what value is the clinical interpretation of lipase?**

Lipases are present in fewer tissues than amylases and for this reason elevations are thought to be more specifically related to pancreatic disease. Inasmuch as serum lipase activity may persist up to a week longer than the serum amylase, a hyperlipasemia is regarded by some to be an invariable sign of acute pancreatic disease.

■ **What other conditions may be associated with elevation of urinary lipase?**

Fat embolization of the lung has been noted to be the cause of increased release of lipase from the injured lung tissue.

■ **Does serum lipase activity correlate with severity of pancreatic disease?**

Good correlation does not usually exist because lipase activity tends to lag behind the rise in serum amylase by approximately 24 hours. The magnitude of increase, however, does tend to parallel that of the amylase. Additionally, abnormal lipase activity can be detected for up to 14 days after the initial onset of acute pancreatitis.

■ **Does mumps cause an elevation of serum lipase activity?**
No.

■ **Is urinary lipase activity considered useful?**

Some authors think that the urinary excretion of lipase is not reliable.

■ **Which enzymes are most likely to be affected physiologically by a normal pregnancy?**

Elevation of alkaline phosphatase may be normally noted during pregnancy. This is principally related to the placental fraction. Additionally, a slow but continual rise in CPK has been observed from 3 to 5 times the normal elevation, occuring in the third trimester, particularly at the time of delivery.

■ **What effects do contraceptive pills have on enzymes?**

Elevations of SGPT have been found to be a sensitive indicator of apparent liver dysfunction when increased sensitivity to the

Pill occurs. This elevation of SGPT may be as much as 2 times that of the SGOT. Peak incidence for elevated enzymes is observed during the second month. The return to normal has been observed within 4 weeks after the drug has been discontinued. This further points out the value of prescreening patients who are to take the Pill prior to the administration of the drug.

■ **Does toxemia in pregnancy affect enzymes?**

Alkaline phosphatase may be elevated. Additionally, acid phosphatase elevations are also noted. In the preeclamptic states the values may be 2 times the nonpregnant level and greater than 65% of that normally seen during the third trimester.

■ **What is the value of performing a ceruloplasmin determination?**

Ceruloplasmin is a copper oxidase that occurs in plasma. Elevations have been noted in association with oral contraceptives and pregnancy; however, its principal clinical use is in diagnosis of Wilson's disease, in which a marked decrease in activity is observed. Other causes for elevations are Hodgkin's disease, hyperthyroidism, and acute inflammatory states.

■ **How many cholinesterases exist?**

Two major cholinesterases exist: the true or type 1, which is an acetocholinesterase, and the pseudo or type 2 cholinesterase.

■ **Where is acetocholinesterase located?**

Acetocholinesterase is found in the erythrocyte and in nerve tissue, particularly at the point of synapse. Pseudocholinesterase is present in the serum.

■ **What is the clinical usefulness for cholinesterase determination?**

A decrease in serum cholinesterase (type 2) is associated with hepatitis, cirrhosis, and carcinoma of the liver. Measurement of the serum erythrocyte cholinesterase of type 1 is valuable in the determination of exposure to organic phosphate insecticides. In such a situation, reduced activity up to 40% may be observed.

■ **Of what further importance is the determination of pseudocholinesterase (type 2)?**

Certain individuals genetically have an altered cholinesterase, referred to as an atypical variant, which cannot hydrolyze succinylcholine. This atypical enzyme may be distinguished from normal pseudocholinesterase because it is not inhibited by either fluoride or dibucaine. Ten possible genetic combinations exist; however, those patients who have a homozygous abnormality will have a low dibucaine number and a low fluoride number.

■ **Where is aldolase located?**

Aldolase is localized principally in the skeletal muscle and in lesser amounts in the heart, liver, and red cells.

■ **In what clinical conditions are elevations of aldolase observed?**

Elevations are primarily observed in muscle disease such as muscular dystrophy and polymyositis; they may also be observed in liver disease and myocardial infarction.

■ **What is the basic structure of a steroid?**

The basic structure of a steroid is a 17-carbon aromatic compound referred to as cyclopentanophenanthrene. To this 17-carbon molecule are added the two angular groups at positions 10 and 13. The angular carbon at position 13 is carbon 18 and the angular carbon added to position 10 is carbon 19. Those carbons added to position 17 are 20 and 21.

■ **What are the androgenic compounds?**

The androgenic compounds are the C-19 compounds. These include the steroids, which have two angular methyl groups, one at C-10 and C-13 and at position 17, rather than having additional carbons has either a keto or hydroxyl group.

■ **What are the estrogenic compounds?**

The estrogenic compounds are C-18 compounds, that is, having only one additional methyl group, at position 13. Additionally, aromatization of the first ring is characteristic of estrogen; that is, the first ring or A-ring is converted into a benzene configuration.

■ **What are the progestational compounds?**

Progestational compounds are C-21 compounds similar to the adrenocorticohormones but having a methyl group at position 21 rather than a hydroxyl, which is characteristic of the adrenocorticoids.

■ **Of the adrenocorticohormones, what are the structural requirements for activity?**

The requirements are: a double bond between positions 4 and 5, a ketone group in position 3, and a ketone group in position 20.

■ **Which radicals impart a specific activity on the adrenocorticoids?**

C-21 hydroxylation enhances sodium retention and is effective in carbohydrate metabolism. C-17 hydroxylated compounds increase carbohydrate activity. This includes hydrocortisone and cortisone.

C-11 oxygenated compounds decrease sodium retention and are also necessary for carbohydrate activity. This group includes corticosterone and dehydrocorticosterone. They inhibit membrane permeability and have an effect on suppressing lymphocytes, eosinophils, and basophils. C-11 deoxygenated compounds (no oxygen) have a profound effect on water and electrolyte metabolism. This group of compounds includes aldosterone.

■ **What is a summary of the total effect of adrenocortical compounds?**

The adrenocortical compounds have an effect on glucose metabolism, causing gluconeogenesis and hyperglycemia. For this reason they are thought to be diabetogenic. Because of the effect on acid mucopolysaccharides and chondroitin sulfate, adrenocortical compounds lead to osteoporosis. The corticoids induce negative nitrogen balance and for that reason are considered catabolic. They tend to promote release of unesterified fatty acids from adipose tissue and are therefore lipemic. They induce lysis of lymph nodes inducing lymphopenia and therefore are considered to be immunosuppressive. Additionally they are anti-inflammatory and have a profound effect on sodium and potassium metabolism.

■ **What is considered to be the common precursor of all steroids?**

Cholesterol is the common precursor of all steroids.

■ **What are the sources of the steroids which are generally determined in the clinical lab?**

Sources of steroids are adrenocorticoids from the adrenal glands, androgens from the testes, and estrogens from the ovaries.

■ **Are estrogen and androgen produced only in the ovary and testis, respectively?**

No. Although estrogens are produced predominantly by the ovary, small amounts are produced by the adrenal gland. Conversely, the androgens are produced predominantly by the testis; however, one-third to one-quarter of the androgens in the form of ketosteroids are produced by the adrenal.

■ **What are 17-ketosteroids?**

17-ketosteroids are that group of compounds having a ketone group at position 17 of the D-ring.

■ **What is the Zimmermann reaction?**

The Zimmermann reaction is that reaction used in the clinical laboratory for determining the level of the 17-ketosteroids.

■ **What is the principal reagent in the Zimmermann reaction?**

The principal reagent is dinitrobenzene in association with methanol and potassium hydroxide.

■ **What is the purpose of the Zimmermann reaction?**

The Zimmermann reaction reflects the activity of adrenal and testicular function. In the male, two-thirds to three-fourths of the 17-ketosteroids are derived from the testes and one-third to one-quarter from the adrenal. In the normal female, the majority of the 17-ketosteroids arise from the adrenal; however, some small amount may arise from the hilar region of the ovary.

■ **What does the Zimmermann reaction measure?**

The Zimmermann reaction measures 17-ketosteroids arising from the adrenal, principally dehydroepiandrosterone and 11-keto-etiocholanolone, and from the testes, androsterone and etiocholanolone. However, most importantly the test does not measure testosterone which is not a 17-ketosteroid, but rather an androgen which has a hydroxyl group at position 17.

■ **What is the clinical significance of elevations of the 17-keto-steroids?**

Increases are noted in adrenocortical carcinoma (particularly in the form of elevated dehydroepiandrosterone), in acromegaly, and in tumors of the testis and masculinizing tumors of the ovary. Decreases are noted in Addison's disease, panhypopituitarism, myxedema, and nephrosis.

■ **What are the Porter-Silber chromogens?**

The Porter-Silber chromogens are the 17-hydroxycorticoids which combine with phenylhydrazine. The phenylhydrazine reacts with the ketone group present at position 20 forming a chromogen when a hydroxyl group is present at positions 17 and 21.

■ **What does the 17-hydroxycorticoid determination measure?**

17-hydroxycorticoid determination measures principally biologically active cortisone, hydrocortisone, and 11-deoxycortisol. The measurement of the corticoids is generally considered to be a better indication of adrenocortical function than the measure of the 17-ketosteroid.

■ **In what clinical situations are there elevations of 17-hydroxy-corticoids?**

Cushing's syndrome, eclampsia, and acute pancreatitis manifest such elevations.

■ **In what clinical situations are the measures of hydroxycorti-coids low?**

In Addison's disease and hypopituitarism the measures are low.

■ **What are the 17-ketogenics?**

The 17-ketogenics include the 17-hydroxycorticoids. Additionally, those compounds having hydroxyl groups on positions 17, 20, and 21, as well as those having a hydroxyl group only on position 17 and the ketone group on position 20 with a methyl group at position 21. These compounds include cortisone, hydrocortisone, 17-hydroxyprogesterone, pregnanetriol, and the tetrahydro derivatives of cortisone, cortisol, and cortexolone.

■ **What is the reaction whereby the 17-ketogenics are determined?**

First is a reduction phase incorporating the use of sodium borohydride, followed by an oxidative phase using sodium bismuthate or periodate forming a 17-keto group. Subsequently a standard Zimmermann reaction is employed utilizing dinitrobenzene.

■ **What are the clinical conditions associated with an elevation of 17-ketogenics?**

The ketogenics are sensitive in the evaluation of the adrenocortical activity and are particularly useful in the diagnosis of the adrenogenital syndrome.

■ **In the synthesis of steroids, what are the major enzymatic steps in the formation of steroids from cholesterol?**

First, the cholesterol is enzymatically converted to progesterone. From that point, two major sequential pathways of enzymatic alterations of the molecule occur. The first is the hydroxylation of the C-17 forming hydroxyprogesterone, followed by the hydroxylation of the C-21 which forms the 17-hydroxyprogesterone, and finally the hydroxylation of the C-11 position forming cortisol. Cortisol is then converted to cortisone. By other pathways, 17-hydroxyprogesterone can form both deoxycorticosterone, corticosterone, and aldosterone, which are the principal sodium- and potassium-controlling substances. Progesterone can also go on to form androstenedione and testosterone, which in turn form the estrogens.

■ **What is the principal stimulator of the adrenal gland?**

Adrenocorticotropic hormone (ACTH) stimulates the adrenal.

■ **What is the principal feedback substance produced by the adrenal gland which tends to turn ACTH off?**

Cortisol is the principal feedback substance.

■ **What happens clinically when cortisol is not produced or is produced in low quantities?**

Unopposed stimulation of the adrenal by ACTH occurs, causing hyperplasia of the gland and elaboration of the alternate pathway metabolites.

■ **Which metabolites occur chiefly in the urine?**

The metabolites which occur in the urine are present in four forms: (1) the biologically active form of the hormones; (2) the biologically inactive form of the hormone; these are principally tetrahydrocorticosterone and tetrahydrocortisone; (3) 17-ketosteroids, which are mainly conjugated; (4) a small amount of pregnanediol and pregnanetriol. Aldosterone is also elaborated in the urine, usually in the inactive form; however, some free and conjugated aldosterone is also excreted.

■ **What are the principal 17-ketosteroids found in the urine?**

Two forms of the 17-ketosteroids are excreted in the urine. They are the alpha ketosteroid, androsterone, and etiocholanolone. Both of these substances are soluble in digitonin. The beta 17-ketosteroids, which include epiandrosterone and dihydroepiandrosterone, are both precipitated by digitonin.

■ **What is the affect of dexamethasone on the Porter-Silber chromogens?**

The Porter-Silber compounds are predominantly cortisol and cortisone. Inasmuch as dexamethasone has an inhibitory effect on ACTH production, the end result is a suppression of the principal 17-hydroxycorticoid, cortisol.

■ **Of what clinical usefulness is the dexamethasone suppression test?**

This test distinguishes between primary and secondary adrenal hyperplasia.

■ **What is the effect of metopirone on steroid metabolism?**

Metopirone is a selective inhibitor of 11-hydroxylation. This substance therefore prevents the formation of cortisol. Consequently, an accumulation of cortisol precursors is measured as 17-hydroxycorticoids in the urine. Without the formation of cortisol, the feedback mechanism for shutting off ACTH production is ineffective. Therefore, in a normal individual metopirone causes an increased stimulation of adrenal activity by causing more ACTH production. This is manifested by an elevation of total ketogenic steroids, a suppression of cortisol, and an elevation of cortisol precursors.

■ **How is the metopirone test used clinically?**

In cases of adrenal hyperplasia, metopirone will cause a two-fold increase in urinary 17-hydroxycorticoids. In carcinoma of the adrenal gland, no change will occur.

■ **What is the effect of dexamethasone on the urinary excretion of 17-hydroxycorticoids?**

In the normal individual dexamethasone suppresses ACTH; therefore the urinary 17-hydroxycorticoids are diminished. In cases of hyperplasia of the adrenal gland caused by increased stimulation by the pituitary, the preadministration values for 17-hydroxycorticoids are elevated and no suppression occurs after administration of low doses of dexamethasone. However, by increasing the dose, effective suppression of hyperplastic glands occurs. This is in counterdistinction to primary tumors of the adrenal gland, which elaborate their own cortisol and thus have already suppressed pituitary ACTH. In that instance, the administration of dexamethasone has no effect.

■ **What is characteristic of the normal physiologic elaboration of 17-hydroxycorticoids?**

A diurnal variation in the elaboration of 17-hydroxycorticoids occurs with approximately 20 μg/dl appearing at 6 AM, which by 6 PM of the same day will fall to approximately half of the morning sample, only to return to the higher fasting level by 6 AM the following day. Characteristically a loss of the diural variation of the level of plasma 17-hydroxycorticoids is indicative of Cushing's syndrome.

■ **What are the four major manifestations of hyperfunction of the adrenal gland?**

The four major manifestations are: (1) increased secretion of all of the adrenocortico hormones as observed in Cushing's syndrome; (2) hypersecretion of androgens, as seen in the adrenogenital syndrome; (3) exclusive hypersecretion of estrogen, as seen in the feminizing syndrome that occurs in male; and (4) exclusive hypersecretion of aldosterone, as observed in primary hyperaldosteronism.

■ **What are the common causes for hyperfunctioning of the adrenal gland?**

The causes of such hyperfunction are (1) pituitary tumor

causing hyperplasia of the adrenal gland, (2) primary hyperplasia of the adrenal gland, and (3) tumors occurring primarily in the adrenal gland. Certain nonendocrine tumors may also produce an ACTH-like substance, e.g., oat-cell carcinoma of the lung.

■ **What are the significant laboratory tests for diagnosing adrenocortical hyperfunction?**

Significant laboratory tests and results include the following: elevation of 17-hydroxycompounds, principally cortisone; elevation of 17-ketosteroids; usually elevation of the 17-ketogenics; and loss of the diural variation in blood cortisol secretion.

■ **What tests are used to distinguish between pituitary tumor, primary adrenal hyperplasia, and tumor of the adrenal gland?**

The suppression tests, principally the dexamethasone suppression test and the metopirone suppression test, are used.

■ **What are the principal causes of hypofunctioning of the adrenal gland (Addison's disease)?**

The principal causes of such hypofunction are: (1) atrophy of the adrenocortex (55% of cases); (2) tuberculosis (approximately 40% of cases); and (3) other causes, including metastatic carcinoma, trauma, and histoplasmosis in approximately 5% of the cases.

■ **Which tests are most likely to be affected by a hypofunctioning adrenal gland?**

Lowered 17-ketosteroids, lowered 17-hyroxycorticoids, and inadequate elevations of 17-hydroxycorticoids after ACTH stimulation will most likely result from such hypofunction.

■ **What controls the function of the anterior pituitary gland?**

The anterior pituitary gland is controlled by regulating hormones produced by the hypothalamus, known as releasing hormones and inhibiting hormones.

■ **Which releasing hormones have been identified?**

Releasing hormone for ACTH, thyrotropin, luteinizing hormone, and follicle stimulating hormone have been isolated, as well as several others.

■ **Have isolated deficiencies in the production of the releasing hormones been described?**

Yes.

■ **How may a diagnosis of hyperfunctioning of the pituitary gland be made on a laboratory basis?**

In the past the determination of hormones elaborated by the

pituitary gland was tedious because these techniques involved bioassay methodology. Radioimmunoassay procedures for follicle stimulating hormone, luteinizing hormone, thyrotropic hormone, growth hormone, and prolactin are currently available. ACTH may also be determined by a radioimmunoassay procedure.

■ **What are some of the common causes for pituitary anterior lobe deficiency?**

The most common causes are pituitary infarction seen in females following pregnancy, destruction of the pituitary by tumor, granuloma, and trauma. The tumors most commonly associated with pituitary deficiencies are chromophobe adenomas and cranial pharyngiomas.

■ **What is the function of the posterior lobe of the pituitary gland?**

The posterior lobe of the pituitary gland acts under direction of osmoreceptors located in the hypothalamus, which respond to changes in blood osmolality. When osmolality levels are high, antidiuretic hormone is released from the hypothalamus and is picked up by capillaries within the posterior pituitary gland. Subsequently, antidiuretic hormone exerts an effect on the distal convoluted tubule of the kidney, causing a reabsorption of water and thus lowering the osmotic pressure.

■ **What disease is associated with faulty production of antidiuretic hormones?**

Diabetes insipidus is associated with faulty production of antidiuretic hormone. The causes for this abnormality include tumor, inflammation, granuloma, trauma, and vascular thrombosis.

■ **What tests are clinically employed to diagnose diabetes insipidus?**

Under constant water loading conditions and using hypertonic saline, nicotine, and vasopressin, the urinary output is measured. If lack of response to these agents is noted, a diagnosis of diabetes insipidus is indicated. However, certain inappropriate responses in ADH production are noted to be associated particularly with hypovolemia following bleeding, edematous states (as noted in cardiac failure), nephrotic syndrome, and cirrhosis. Additionally, certain malignant tumors, particularly of the lung, are associated with inappropriate ADH release.

■ **What are the laboratory manifestations of primary hyperaldosteronism?**

Low serum potassium associated with excessive urinary loss of both potassium and hydrogen ions (hypokalemic alkalosis) is accompanied by an increased serum sodium and increased water reabsorption. This results in hypernatremia and hypervolemia, usually without manifestation of edema.

■ **Which two clinical tests most characterize primary hyperaldosteronism?**

The two tests are: (1) increased urinary excretion of aldosterone; and (2) depressed elaboration of plasma renin.

■ **How is the hypertension associated with hyperaldosteronism differentiated from the hypertension caused by renal vascular disease (secondary hyperaldosteronism)?**

In renal vascular disease, renin (an enzyme elaborated by the kidney and which converts angiotensinogen to angiotensin 1) is elevated, whereas in primary hyperaldosteronism the renin activity is very low.

■ **What is Bartter's syndrome?**

Bartter's syndrome is characterized by high aldosterone, high plasma renin activity, and normal blood pressure.

■ **What are the characteristics of infantile adrenogenital syndrome?**

In infantile adrenogenital syndrome, simple virilism is caused by faulty biosynthesis of the adrenocorticosteroids. This results principally from an enzymatic block in hydroxylation of the cortisol precursors. With a deficiency of cortisol and unopposed elaboration of ACTH, adrenal hyperplasia occurs and is predominantly manifested by masculinization of the external genitalia of female infants.

■ **What is the most common enzymatic block responsible for infantile adrenogenital syndrome?**

The block of 21-hydroxylation is the most common.

■ **Is the adrenogenital syndrome noted in adults?**

Yes. The cause of adrenogenital syndrome in adults may also be selective enzymatic blocks in production of cortisol; however, it may be associated with adenomas or carcinoma. In the event that it occurs in a female, evidence of excessive 17-ketosteroid production is noted associated with clinical evidence of masculinization. The urinary 17-ketosteroids are only moderately elevated in hyperplasias of a benign order, but may be markedly elevated in cases of adenoma and adenocarcinoma.

■ **What is the function of the adrenal medulla?**

The medullary portion of the adrenal gland produces substances that are responsible for the clinical sign of fight or flight, i.e., sweating, rapid pulse rate, increase of blood pressure, flushing face, dilated pupils, and loss of visceral function.

■ **What are the principal substances emanating from the adrenal medulla found in the urine?**

Epinephrine, norepinephrine, metanephrine, normetanephrine, and vanilmandelic acid are found in urine.

■ **What are the principal metabolites of the adrenal medulla found in the urine?**

The composition is the following: (1) free vanilmandelic acid, approximately 40%; (2) conjugated and free metanephrine associated with conjugated and free normetanephrine, 40%; (3) the combined catecholamines, epinephrine, and norepinephrine, the remaining 20%. The ratio of epinephrine to norepinephrine is approximately 1:4.

■ **What is the clinical significance of elevation of these catecholamines?**

In association with a tumor of the adrenal medulla (referred to as pheochromocytoma), elevations of the catecholamines occur. Those tumors arising from the adrenal gland proper tend to secrete norepinephrine and epinephrine, whereas those tumors arising outside of the adrenal predominantly tend to produce norepinephrine.

■ **What other tests are employed in the diagnosis of pheochromocytoma?**

The provocative histamine test is used during a lull in the hypertension that is usually associated with the disease. Also, a regitine test is sometimes used when the patient is hypertensive.

■ **Should any precautions be taken before performing a laboratory evaluation for the elaboration of vanilmandelic acid?**

Yes. Vanilla and products containing vanilla extracts, as well as bananas and cocoa, are to be avoided in the diet.

■ **What is the function of the thyroid gland?**

The thyroid gland synthesizes, stores, and secretes thyroid hormone under stimulation by the pituitary gland.

■ **What is the basic physiology involved in the thyroid hormone synthesis?**

Inorganic iodide is absorbed by the gastrointestinal tract and circulates as iodide either to be trapped by the thyroid gland or to be excreted via the salivary gland or urinary tract. The thyrotropic hormone emanating from the pituitary gland enhances the trapping of iodide by the gland, while substances such as thiocyanate can block this activity. In the thyroid cells the iodide is converted by an oxidative enzyme into iodine. This activity can be blocked by thiouracil. The oxidized iodine is then rapidly utilized in the iodination of tyrosine to form mono- and diiodotyrosine. Sulfonamide derivatives interfere with the iodination of tyrosine. The combination of the mono- and diiodinated tyrosine results in the formation of thyroxine (T4) and of triiodothyronine (T3). These substances are then stored in the gland in a large molecular form known as thyroglobulin.

■ **How are the thyroid hormones released from the gland?**

The hormones T3 and T4 are released from thyroglobulin by proteolytic enzymes. The hormones are then transported to the peripheral tissue by thyroxine-binding proteins that are present in the serum.

■ **Where is the major thyroxine binding protein located?**

The binding protein is located between the alpha-1 and alpha-2 globulins; this globulin is known as an interalpha globulin.

■ **Which of the hormones is the most biologically active?**

Although T4 is present quantitatively in larger amounts in the serum, T3 is the most active of the two.

■ **What is the feedback to the pituitary gland that inhibits TSH production?**

Thyroxine (T4) is the principal substance that inhibits the release of TSH.

■ **Can globulins other than the interalpha globulin bind the thyroid hormones?**

Yes. Thyroxine can also bind to prealbumin and to a lesser degree to albumin. Triiodothyronine can bind to albumin; however, it does not bind to prealbumin.

■ **What are the clinical laboratory manifestations of hyperthyroidism?**

The manifestations are: an elevation of the T4; an elevation of the T3; cholesterol normal or low; phospholipids that are lowered; and a low uric acid. There may be an elevation in blood sugar which can produce a diabetic tolerance curve, and there may be a relative lymphocytosis.

■ **Is the determination of thyroid stimulating hormone (TSH) valuable in diagnosing hyperthyroidism?**

Not usually. It is generally accepted that the TSH should be low; however, the test is more significant when making a diagnosis of hypothyroidism.

■ **Are there substances which can interfere with the thyroid test?**

Interference of thyroid tests depends upon the methodology employed. If the competitive binding analysis for serum thyroxine is performed, there is little or no interference by inorganic or organic iodides. This problem is present when measurements of thyroid activity are performed by using direct chemical measurements.

■ **Does an elevated or low value of serum total thyroxine always mean increased or decreased production of thyroid hormone?**

No. Alteration in the level of the thyroxine binding globulin will alter the value for serum T4. If a serum-free thyroxine is performed (FT4), variations in TBG will not affect the final result.

■ **Can the binding capacity of thyroid binding globulin and thyroid binding prealbumin be altered?**

Yes. Estrogens and estrogen containing oral contraceptives can cause elevations of the thyroid binding globulin. Conversely, salicylates and Dilantin tend to displace the hormone from the globulin by competition.

■ **What is the effect on the T3-by-column caused by alterations in the thyroid binding globulin?**

Triiodothyronine uptake varies inversely to the amount of thyroid binding protein available. When there is an increase in binding protein, as seen in pregnancy, the T3 values will be lower. When the protein levels are low, the T3 test will be elevated.

■ **What laboratory test of thyroid function circumvents the effect of protein alteration?**

The determination of free thyroxine circumvents the effects of altered protein concentration.

■ **Is the determination of ^{131}I uptake by the thyroid an effective test?**

The ^{131}I tracer uptake continues to be helpful in distinguishing thyroid hyperfunction from normal function; however, it is inadequate to distinguish euthyroid states from hypothyroid states. It is also useful in assisting in the diagnosis of thyroiditis.

■ **By what method may the thyroid stimulating hormone be evaluated?**

The determination of thyroid stimulating hormone by radioimmunoassay is the most sensitive method. It is used to distinguish between primary hypothyroidism caused by primary thyroid failure and secondary hypothyroidism caused by pituitary failure. The serum TSH is elevated in the former and is low or absent in the latter.

■ **What is LATS?**

LATS is long-acting thyroid stimulator. It is an immunoglobulin produced by lymphocytes and is found in the serum of patients with Graves' disease.

■ **What tests are useful in monitoring a patient who is getting replacement therapy for a hypofunctioning thyroid gland?**

There is evidence to suggest that T4 is converted peripherally to T3. Consequently, methods for T4 determination are inadequate in that circulating T3 is not measured by the usual techniques for measuring T4. Therefore the patient may be euthyroid (normal) while taking T3 and still have a low serum total T4 and free T4. Generally, patients who take desiccated thyroid frequently have a low normal or slightly decreased serum total T4, whereas patients taking a mixture of T3 and T4 have a serum total T4 within the normal range. Some believe that the best guide is the determination of serum thyroid stimulating hormone, which will be in the normal range if the patient is receiving adequate therapy and elevated if not.

■ **What is T3 toxicosis?**

T3 toxicosis, a variant of Graves' disease, is characterized by a normal or low serum T4, an elevated T3, and a normal thyroid binding globulin. This is associated with an elevated or normal ^{131}I uptake by the thyroid gland, which cannot be suppressed when T3 is administered.

■ **What is calcitonin?**

Calcitonin is a polypeptide produced by the parafollicular cells of the thyroid which cause hypocalcemia. Similar cells are observed in the thymus and parathyroid gland.

■ **What is the effect of calcitonin on the human body?**

Calcitonin decreases bone resorption, increases urinary excretion of calcium and phosphorus, and induces hypocalcemia and hypophosphatemia.

■ **In what situation is there an elevation of calcitonin?**

In medullary carcinoma of the thyroid, elevations of calcitonin are known. Additionally, when medullary carcinoma of the thyroid exists, there may be associated hyperparathyroidism, multiple tumors of the adrenal medulla (pheochromocytoma), and tumors of the mucous membrane (ganglioneuroma).

■ **What is myxedema?**

Myxedema is a disease caused by hypofunctioning of the thyroid gland. It is characterized by low T4, low T3, low ^{131}I uptake, elevated cholesterol, low 17-ketosteroid, and low BMR.

■ **What are the causes of myxedema?**

Myxedema may be caused primarily by failure of the thyroid to produce hormones, or it may be secondary to pituitary hypofunctioning.

■ **How can one distinguish between primary myxedema and secondary myxedema?**

In primary myxedema, TSH values are high and values for T3 and T4 cannot be elevated after the administration of additional TSH. In secondary myxedema, T3 and T4 levels may be elevated after the administration of TSH.

■ **Can hypothyroidism occur in infants?**

Yes. Cretinism is the result of congenital absence of the thyroid hormone, or it may be associated with nonfunctioning goiters or goiters incapable of synthesizing normal hormones.

■ **What is hypoparathyroidism?**

It is a disease caused by deficiency of parathormone, most commonly seen following subtotal or total thyroidectomy.

■ **What is the chemical picture of hypoparathyroidism?**

The findings are a low serum calcium associated with a high serum phosphorus and a low excretion of calcium and phosphorus in the urine associated with a normal alkaline phosphatase.

■ **What is hyperparathyroidism?**

Hyperparathyroidism is a diseased state in which there is an overproduction of parathormone caused primarily by hyperplasia or adenoma of the parathyroid. It may be caused secondarily by chronic renal insufficiency.

■ **How is the laboratory diagnosis of hyperparathyroidism made?**

The presence of elevated serum calcium with associated low serum phosphate, increased amounts of calcium and phosphate in the urine, and increases in serum alkaline phosphatase indicates hyperparathyroidism. When associated with an elevated calcium, the single best indication of hyperparathyroidism is an elevated parathormone. Elevations of proline and hydroxyproline and cyclic AMP in the urine are other manifestations of hyperparathyroidism.

■ **How can primary hyperparathyroidism be distinguished from secondary hyperparathyroidism?**

In hyperparathyroidism caused by renal disease, the parathormone levels will be elevated but the serum calcium level will be in the normal range, whereas in primary hyperparathyroidism the parathormone and calcium levels are both elevated.

■ **Is hyperparathyroidism the only disease entity that can cause an elevated calcium?**

No. Elevated serum calciums may be seen in the milk-alkali syndrome, vitamin D intoxication, sarcoidosis, multiple myeloma, metastatic carcinoma usually involving bone, thyrotoxicosis, and disuse atrophy or osteoparosis. In these instances, however, the serum calcium is elevated but the parathormone levels are low.

■ **In polycystic disease of the ovary (Stein-Leventhal) what laboratory determinations are helpful in diagnosing this disease entity?**

High plasma luteinizing hormone levels, associated with unusually low follicle stimulating hormone levels, are associated with polycystic disease. This results from the fact that in the polycystic ovary syndrome, estrogen secretion is maintained and inhibits pituitary FSH.

■ **Can endocrine syndromes be caused by cancer of nonendocrine organs?**

Yes. Gonadotropin-like hormone has been measured in patients with lung cancer of all types. Human chorionic gonadotropin-like hormone has been recorded in association with carcinoma of the lung, liver, breast, and renal cell and with malignant melanoma. ACTH-like hormone has been reported most commonly with oat-cell tumors of the bronchus, but has also been seen with tumors of the thymus and pancreas. TSH-like hormone has been associated with trophoblastic tumors and tumors of the testes. Parathyroid-like hormone has been detected with lung cancer, kidney cancer, and cancers of the uterus, ovary, and GI tract.

ELECTROLYTES

GORDON LANG

JOAN SHROUT

■ Discuss the distribution of water in the human body.

Water comprises approximately 50 to 70% of the weight of the body. The percentage varies inversely with the amount of adipose tissue present and is located in several compartments. (1) Intracellular fluid—30 to 35% of the body weight or 55% of the total body water is located within the cells. (2) Extracellular fluid —25 to 30% of the body weight or 45% of the total body water is located outside of the cells. The extracellular fluid is located in several subcompartments: (a) plasma water—about 4.5% of body weight; (b) interstitial fluid and lymph—about 12% of body weight; (c) dense connective tissue, cartilage, and bone water— about 9% of body weight; and (d) transcellular water—about 1.5% of body weight. This is water formed by the secretory cells of the gastrointestinal and respiratory tracts, skin, kidney, brain, thyroid, and gonads.

Water is dynamic as it moves from one compartment to another. Dehydration and water overload are reflected in all compartments.

■ Discuss the sources of body water and the routes of normal and abnormal water loss.

The major source of water is that ingested by the oral route. This normally amounts to 1,500 to 3,000 ml per day. A second source is water obtained from oxidation of foodstuff. The oxidation of each 100 calories of a mixed diet generates 12 ml of water. Oxidation of body tissues is a fluid source that produces about 300 to 400 ml per day.

Water loss is divided into sensible and insensible loss. The normal daily sensible loss consists of about 15 ml of urine per kilogram of body weight and 100 ml of fecal water. The normal insensible loss from the lungs and skin amounts daily to about 15 ml of water per kilogram of body weight.

Abnormal losses of water occur in periods of increased activity and during certain disease states. Normally about 8,000 ml of digestive juices are secreted into the gastrointestinal tract and all but 100 ml are reabsorbed. Abnormal losses of gastrointestinal fluid occur in conditions that result in diarrhea and vomiting or after gastrointestinal drainage procedures. An abnormal amount of in-

Holmes' formula can be used to calculate osmolality of blood.

$$mOsm/kg = 1.86 \times Na \ (mEq/L) + \frac{Glucose \ (mg/dl)}{18} + \frac{Urea \ nitrogen \ (mg/dl)}{2.8}$$

1.86 represents the osmotic coefficient for sodium chloride, 18 represents the molecular weight of glucose, and 2.8 represents the molecular weight of urea nitrogen.

In order to calculate the osmolality, the values for sodium, glucose, and urea nitrogen must be known, as indicated by the above formula. In addition to these three substances, chloride, bicarbonate and phosphate also contribute significantly to the osmolality and are accounted for by the osmotic coefficient 1.86.

Protein contributes little to total osmolality. To calculate the concentration of protein as mOsm/kg of plasma water, the concentration of protein (gm/dl) is divided by 8. For example, a protein of 8.6 gm/dl is equal to 1.075 mOsm/kg.

Using Holmes' formula, the calculated osmolality is usually 5 to 8 mOsm/kg lower than the measured osmolality. A measured osmolality which greatly exceeds the calculated value indicates serious illness characterized by elevation of unmeasured solute (e.g., lactic acid, medications, alcohol, etc.).

■ **Discuss the clinical value of osmolality.**

The distribution of water between the various fluid compartments is regulated by their osmolality. Hypertonicity of serum will result in cellular dehydration and dilution of the serum by cellular water. Hypotonicity of serum will result in cellular hydration and edema.

The measurement of osmolality is useful in the evaluation of fluid and electrolyte abnormalities such as the differentiation of the causes of hyponatremia and hypernatremia. The concentrating ability of the kidney is best measured utilizing the urine osmolality rather than specific gravity determinations.

The ratio of urine/serum osmolality is useful in the evaluation of the polyurias and the inappropriate secretion of antidiuretic hormone syndrome.

■ **Define and discuss hypokalemia.**

Potassium is the most important intracellular cation. About 98% of the body potassium is located in the intracellular space. It is also present within the extracellular fluid. The normal plasma concentration is 3.5 to 5.5 mEq/L plasma. Potassium and sodium help maintain a normal distribution of body water and normal intracellular enzymatic and metabolic reactions.

A plasma potassium concentration of less than 3.5 mEq/L is known as hypokalemia. A deficit of potassium may be present and not be reflected as a low plasma potassium concentration in some states of hemoconcentration and acidosis. Plasma potassium levels must be interpreted with knowledge of the blood pH. During acidosis, potassium shifts from the intracellular space to the extracellular space and the hydrogen ion shifts from the extracellular space to to the intracellular space. Generally, plasma potassium concentration rises 0.6 mEq/L for each 0.1 unit fall in blood pH. Acidosis is therefore associated with an intracellular potassium deficiency and increase in extracellular potassium.

The kidneys have the ability to conserve sodium and to produce sodium-free urine. They do not, however, have the ability to conserve potassium. When potassium intake is eliminated or significantly reduced, potassium depletion results because from 20 to 60 mEq/L/24 hours is eliminated in the urine.

Hypokalemia secondary to an increased renal excretion of potassium occurs in conditions of bicarbonate excess (metabolic alkalosis). Excessive administration of adrenal cortical steroids and hyperaldosteronism result in an increased potassium excretion and concomitant potassium depletion.

Clinical conditions associated with hypokalemia

1. Abnormal urinary loss of potassium
    a. Overadministration of adrenal cortical steroids
    b. Prolonged diuretic therapy (one of the most common causes)
    c. Primary aldosteronism
    d. Cushing's disease
    e. Renal tubular acidosis (inability of renal tubules to maintain a hydrogen ion gradient across the tubular membrane with substitution of potassium for the hydrogen ion in the sodium reabsorption exchange mechanisms)
    f. Diabetic ketoacidosis (occurs following correction of acidosis without administration of potassium)
    g. Respiratory acidosis
    h. Hepatic insufficiency
    i. Starvation and malnutrition
2. Abnormal gastrointestinal loss
    a. Vomiting
    b. Malabsorption syndromes
    c. Diarrhea

d. Enemas
3. Shift of potassium from serum to cells
   a. Periodic familial paralysis (a rare condition with intermittent attacks of skeletal muscle paralysis)
   b. Extracorporeal perfusion (cardiopulmonary bypass)

■ **Define and indicate some clinical causes for hyperkalemia.**

A plasma potassium concentration of more than 5.5 mEq/L is known as hyperkalemia. Inadequate renal excretion of potassium is the most frequent cause of hyperkalemia. This occurs during oliguria or anuria in acute and chronic renal failure of almost any etiology. Decreased potassium excretion and hyperkalemia also occur in adrenal insufficiency (Addison's disease). As discussed earlier, hyperkalemia may be present in conditions of severe acidosis. Hyperkalemia has been reported in a condition known as malignant hyperthermia, which is hyperpyrexia associated with the administration of various anesthetic agents and the muscle relaxant succinylcholine.

Pseudohyperkalemia is present in certain individuals with thrombocytosis. This is an artificial elevation of serum potassium caused by the release of potassium from platelets during the clotting process. This can be avoided by using only heparinized plasma for electrolyte determinations. Hemolysis will falsely elevate plasma potassium as will prolonged contact of plasma with the red cells.

■ **Define and discuss hyponatremia.**

Sodium is the most important cation of the extracellular fluid space; its concentration exceeds that of all of the other cations. The normal plasma sodium concentration is 135 to 145 mEq/L. Sodium is present in a much lower concentration within the intracellular fluid. Sodium is important in the maintenance of normal water distribution. Along with chloride and bicarbonate, it regulates acid-base metabolism. Sodium also functions to maintain normal neuromuscular irritability.

Hyponatremia is a condition in which the plasma sodium concentration is less than 130 mEq/L. A reduction in the plasma sodium results in a lowering of the osmolality. This inhibits the secretion of antidiuretic hormone (ADH) from the posterior pituitary gland causing excretion of water, resulting in an increase in the plasma sodium concentration. Hypernatremia, conversely, results in an increase in plasma osmolality resulting in a release of ADH which promotes retention of water. Generally, hyponatremia results from an excessive amount of water intake, a loss of sodium without a proportional loss of water, or internal shifts of water and electrolytes.

Clinical conditions associated with hyponatremia

I. Pseudohyponatremia
   A. Laboratory error—quality control measures should eliminate most of this type
   B. Displacement of water. Electrolytes are normally performed on plasma, the water content of which varies from 91 to 93%. This percentage may be significantly reduced whenever hyperlipemia or hyperproteinemia is present. As sodium concentration is expressed as mEq/L of plasma and not mEq/L of plasma water, the sodium concentration will be reduced. A normal sodium concentration in a grossly lipemic plasma is an elevated sodium. The plasma osmolality is normal in this type of hyponatremia.

II. Dilutional hyponatremia
   A. Water excess
      1. Exogenous (acute—self-inflicted or iatrogenic; intravenous fluids, enemas, etc.)
      2. Endogenous
         a. Inappropriate secretion of antidiuretic hormone (ADH) features:
            (1) Hyponatremia and low serum osmolality
            (2) Hypertonic urine that may contain considerable amounts of sodium
            (3) Absence of azotemia (normal renal function)
            (4) Normal blood volume so that antidiuresis is not being stimulated by extracellular volume depletion
            (5) Hyponatremia and hypernaturia corrected following fluid restriction
            (6) Occurs:
               (a) Postoperatively in the elderly
               (b) In patients with certain malignant tumors that occasionally secrete ADH-like substances (lung, duodenum, pancreas)
               (c) In certain central nervous system disorders
               (d) In diseases of the lung (pneumonia, TB)
         b. Idiopathic—present in long-standing heart or liver failure, probably related to excessive renal proximal reabsorption of water
   B. Accumulation of nonelectrolyte solutes in the extracellular fluid (hyperosmolality). The accumulation of glucose and/or urea nitrogen in the extracellular fluid results in an osmotic gradient between the cells and the interstitial fluid. This gradient results in a shift of water from the intracellular to the extracellular compartment resulting in hyponatremia and overall dilution of the hyperosmolar extracellular fluid. Each 35 mg/dl rise in extracellular glu-

cose and each 5 mg/dl rise in urea nitrogen results in a 1 mEq/L fall in extracellular fluid (plasma) sodium. This type of hyponatremia is seen in uncontrolled diabetes mellitus and azotemic states.

C. True sodium depletion—hyponatremia caused by sodium loss occurs following:
   1. Renal loss—osmotic diuresis, following diuretic therapy, in renal disease, in adrenal insufficiency
   2. Gastrointestinal loss—vomiting, diarrhea, nasogastric suction
   3. Cutaneous loss—perspiration (excessive), burns
   4. Loss of body fluids secondary to thoracentesis or paracentesis
   5. Hemorrhage

■ **Define and discuss hypernatremia.**

Hypernatremia is a condition in which the plasma sodium is greater than 150 mEq/L of plasma. It usually results from an inadequate intake of water or excessive water loss. The hypernatremia leads to hyperosmolar states that result in cellular dehydration.

Hypernatremia occurs following deficient water intake, an excessive output of water such as occurs in diabetes insipidus, protracted vomiting or diarrhea, and cerebral trauma with loss of ADH control. It may also occur iatrogenically following excess administration of hypertonic sodium chloride solutions.

■ **Discuss chloride shift.**

Hemoglobin is one of the important buffers responsible for the maintenance of a normal blood pH. Oxyhemoglobin (HbO) is a stronger acid than reduced hemoglobin (HHb). The formation of HbO from HHb within the erythrocytes located in the lungs results in the release of H^+ which reacts with HCO_3^- to form carbonic acid (H_2CO_3). Under the influence of carbonic anhydrase, the H_2CO_3 is converted to H_2O and CO_2. The latter is released to the alveolar air and expired. At this same time HCO_3^- from the plasma enters the erythrocyte. Chloride, in response, shifts from the erythrocyte to the plasma (the so called chloride shift).

HHb is formed from HbO upon release of O_2 to the tissues. CO_2 produced in the tissues enters the erythrocytes where under the influence of the enzyme carbonic anhydrase H_2CO_3 is formed. The latter is ionized to form H^+ and HCO_3^-. The reduced Hb reacts with the H^+ to form HHb. Some of the HCO_3^- that is formed enters the plasma, which results in a shift in the chloride from the plasma to the erythrocyte. Therefore arterial plasma has a higher chloride than does venous plasma.

■ **What is an acid? What is a base?**

According to the Brönsted theory an acid is a proton (hydrogen ion, H^+) donor. A base is a proton accepter.

$$H_2CO_3 \rightleftharpoons HCO_3^- + H^+$$

Acid   Base

■ **What is an anion? What is a cation?**

An anion is a negatively charged ion, e.g., Cl^-, which migrates in an electrical field to the anode. A cation is a positively charged ion, e.g., Na^+, which migrates in an electrical field to the cathode.

■ **Define pH.**

pH is a simplified expression of hydrogen ion concentration and is equal to the negative logarithm of the hydrogen ion concentration. A decreasing pH represents an increasing H^+ concentration. A 0.3 unit fall in the pH is equivalent to a doubling of the H^+ concentration.

pH	$[H^+]$
7.10	80 nM/L
7.40	40 nM/L
7.70	20 nM/L

The normal ranges are 7.32 to 7.42 (venous) and 7.35 to 7.45 (arterial).

■ **Define P_{CO_2}.**

P_{CO_2} is the partial pressure of CO_2 in a gas phase in equilibrium with liquid blood. It is a measurement of respiratory function, indicating the adequacy of ventilation. The term "hypercapnia" indicates hypoventilation, resulting in an elevated P_{CO_2}. Hypocapnia indicates hyperventilation, resulting in a low P_{CO_2}. The normal P_{CO_2} ranges are 42 to 55 torr (venous) and 34 to 46 torr (arterial).

■ **What is the Henderson-Hasselbalch equation?**

The Henderson-Hasselbalch equation is an expression of the fundamental relation of physiologic acid-base chemistry, and is written as follows:

$$pH = pK + \log \frac{base}{acid} \qquad (1)$$

For the carbonic acid–bicarbonate system it is written:

$$pH = 6.1 + \log \frac{[HCO_3^-] \ mEq/L}{[H_2CO_3] \ mEq/L} \qquad (2)$$

where

$6.1 = pK$ of H_2CO_3 at $38°$ C. in serum

pH should be thought of as simply the ratio of $[HCO_3^-]$: $[H_2CO_3]$. The pH is directly proportional to this ratio. For example, the ratio resulting in a pH of 7.40 is 20:1.

If any two of the parameters pH, $[HCO_3^-]$, or $[H_2CO_3]$ are known, the third parameter can be readily calculated. The $[H_2CO_3]$ is obtainable from the Pco_2, as the $[H_2CO_3]$ is directly proportional to the Pco_2.

$$[H_2CO_3] = 0.03 \times Pco_2 \qquad (3)$$

where

0.03 = solubility coefficient of CO_2 at 37° C. relating $[H_2CO_3]$ to Pco_2

The availability of direct measurements of pH and Pco_2 and the above equation allow for the calculation of other parameters, HCO_3^-, H_2CO_3, and total CO_2. Nomograms of Siggaard-Anderson and Weisberg, or the utilization of minicomputers such as those produced by Olivetti, Wang, and others, simplify the calculation.

■ **Define buffer base.**

Buffer base is the sum of the concentrations in mEq/L of the buffer anions of whole blood: bicarbonate, phosphate, hemoglobin, and plasma protein. The normal range is 46 to 50 mEq/L.

■ **Define base excess (BE).**

Base excess is equal to the actual buffer base minus the normal buffer base (defined above). The actual determination of BE is not practical, but it can readily be determined using the Siggaard-Anderson alignment nomogram when the pH, Pco_2, and hemoglobin are known. If a programable calculator is available, BE can also be calculated using the equation of Alvin P. Long, Jr.

$$BE = \left[1 - \frac{Hb}{75}\right] [HCO_3^-] - 23.94 + [11.4 + 1.323\ Hb]\ [pH - 7.4]$$

The normal range is −2.5 to +2.5 mEq/L.

For practical purposes, BE is a measurement of bicarbonate excess or deficit. A positive result indicates metabolic alkalosis (bicarbonate excess) and a negative value below the normal range indicates metabolic acidosis (bicarbonate deficit).

■ **List and define several terms that have been used to describe CO_2.**

Total CO_2 or CO_2 content represents the sum of the bicarbonate, carbonic acid, and the dissolved carbon dioxide that is present in blood drawn anaerobically and at the Pco_2 present in vivo. Total

CO_2 can be best determined by calculation utilizing the Henderson-Hasselbalch equation when pH and Pco_2 are known. Direct measurements utilizing the Van Slyke blood gas apparatus or the Natelson microgasometer have been performed in the past prior to the advent of modern blood gas analyzers.

CO_2 combining power and *CO_2 capacity* measure the carbon dioxide of separated or true plasma following equilibration to a Pco_2 of 40 torr. After correcting for dissolved CO_2 (i.e., H_2CO_3), it represents bicarbonate. These parameters are only of historical interest.

Bicarbonate is the $[HCO_3^-]$ in anaerobically drawn blood and is best determined by calculation utilizing the Henderson-Hasselbalch equation.

Standard bicarbonate was defined by Jorgensen and Astrup as the plasma bicarbonate concentration in fully oxygenated blood at $38°$ C when the Pco_2 is 40 torr. This parameter was popular prior to the development of the direct Pco_2 electrode and was derived utilizing the Astrup method and apparatus.

■ **What is the minimum data required to adequately evaluate a clinical acid-base disorder?**

A pH, Pco_2, and HCO_3^- is the minimum data necessary to adequately evaluate and manage a clinical acid base disorder. "CO_2" by whatever method, without a pH and Pco_2, is insufficient, not only to evaluate an acid base disorder, but may not uncover a disorder when it exists. A "normal" total CO_2 content of 27 mEq/L can occur with a pH of 6.80, 7.80, or anywhere in between. This is analogous to informing a visitor to Washington, D. C. that the White House is on Pennsylvania Avenue with the result that he arrives at the Capitol or at the I.R.S. Office. It is essential to provide routine pH, Pco_2, and HCO_3^- measurements on all requests for "CO_2." It is valid to perform these determinations under all circumstances on properly drawn venous blood.

■ **How is blood pH and Pco_2 measured?**

pH or $[H^+]$ is determined potentiometrically by a hydrogen ion permeable glass electrode which contains an Ag/AgCl wire immersed in an electrolyte of fixed pH. An electrical potential is created when a glass membrane separates two solutions of different $[H^+]$. This potential is compared to a reference voltage supplied by a Hg/Hg_2Cl_2 (calomel) electrode which is connected to the unknown and the glass electrode by a solution of saturated KCl. The membrane potential is proportional to the log $[H^+]$.

P_{CO_2} is also measured potentiometrically. The P_{CO_2} electrode is a combination pH/reference electrode which is covered with a membrane that is permeable to nonionized molecules such as CO_2 gas but not to ions such as $[H^+]$. A thin layer of a bicarbonate solution is located between the membrane and the electrode. The pH of the bicarbonate solution changes in response to CO_2 which diffuses into it from the sample being measured. The change in pH of the bicarbonate solution is exponentially related to the P_{CO_2} of the sample being measured.

■ **Discuss the four types of acid-base imbalance.**

Acid-base disturbances are best described by indicating the alteration in the $[HCO_3^-]:[H_2CO_3]$ ratio. Traditionally, abnormalities in the $[HCO_3^-]$ have been called metabolic and abnormalities in the $[H_2CO_3]$ have been called respiratory. The metabolic component $[HCO_3^-]$ is regulated primarily by renal mechanisms, whereas the respiratory component, P_{CO_2}, is regulated by the lungs. Renal and pulmonary mechanisms attempt to maintain a 20:1 bicarbonate–carbonic acid ratio, by retaining or eliminating HCO_3^- or H_2CO_3 (P_{CO_2}), respectively.

Bicarbonate excess or metabolic alkalosis is a disorder in which the concentration of bicarbonate is increased resulting in an increase in the bicarbonate–carbonic acid ratio. The decrease in $[H^+]$ results in hypoventilation and an increase in the P_{CO_2} ($[H_2CO_3]$). Renal mechanisms are also stimulated to increase bicarbonate excretion, resulting in a lowering of the $[HCO_3^-]$. Common causes for this disorder are vomiting, loss of gastric acid by suction, administration of various diuretic agents, hypokalemia of any etiology, and overadministration of alkali such as sodium bicarbonate.

Bicarbonate deficit or metabolic acidosis is a disorder in which the concentration of bicarbonate is decreased, resulting in a decrease in the bicarbonate–carbonic acid ratio. The increase in $[H^+]$ results in hyperventilation and a decrease in the P_{CO_2} ($[H_2CO_3]$). Renal mechanisms are also activated so as to retain HCO_3^-. Common causes for this disorder are diabetes mellitus, lactic acidosis, salicylate intoxication (late), renal failure, and overadministration of acidifying agents such as NH_4Cl.

Carbonic acid excess or respiratory acidosis is a hypoventilatory disorder in which the concentration of carbonic acid is increased (↑P_{CO_2}), resulting in a decrease in the bicarbonate–carbonic acid ratio. Compensatory renal mechanisms are slowly activated in response to the increased P_{CO_2}, resulting in retention of HCO_3^-. Secondarily, ventilation is increased in response to an elevated P_{CO_2} and a decreased pH. Common causes of hypoventilation are central nervous system depression of any etiology, such as CNS trauma, and use of certain drugs; acute mechanical obstruction of the airway; and chronic obstructive pulmonary disease.

Carbonic acid deficit or respiratory alkalosis is a hyperventilatory disorder in which the concentration of carbonic acid is decreased ($\downarrow P_{CO_2}$), resulting in an increase in the bicarbonate–carbonic acid ratio. Compensation is generally slow unless the cause is alleviated. While there is some increase in renal excretion of bicarbonate following prolonged hyperventilation, a considerable proportion of the lowered HCO_3^- is secondary to a lactic acidosis which occurs as a result of tissue hypoxia. The hypoxia is secondary to a shift to the left in the oxygen dissociation curve which occurs following a rise in pH. Common causes are psychogenic hyperventilation, respiratory center stimulation such as occurs early in salicylate intoxication, fever, and anoxia, hepatic failure, and iatrogenic, secondary to mechanical hyperventilation.

It should be remembered that compensation for an acid-base disorder only occurs if the organ (lung or kidney) responsible is functionally able to respond to the primary disorder. When compensation cannot occur, the patient is in jeopardy.

■ **Discuss the composition of atmospheric air.**

The total pressure exerted by a gas mixture such as atmospheric air is simply the sum of the partial pressure of all of the gases present in the mixture. The barometric pressure (BP) at sea level is about 760 torr. The barometric pressure decreases with altitude: at 18,000 feet it is one-half of that at sea level. Dry atmospheric air contains 20.93% oxygen, 0.03% carbon dioxide, 79.4% nitrogen, and traces of gases such as argon. The percent composition is the same at all altitudes. To calculate the partial pressure of various gases, the percent is multiplied by the barometric pressure.

Air that enters the respiratory tree is rapidly saturated with water vapor, which exerts a partial pressure of 47 torr at 37° C. (The symbol for partial pressure is capital P followed by the gas being discussed.) Therefore, dry atmospheric air at sea level will have a BP of 760-47 or 713 torr.

The partial pressures of dry atmospheric air as it enters the respiratory tree are:

$$P_{O_2} = 0.2093 \times 713 = 149 \text{ torr}$$
$$P_{CO_2} = 0.003 \times 713 = 0.2 \text{ torr}$$
$$P_{N_2} = 0.7904 \times 713 = 564 \text{ torr}$$

■ **Discuss the composition of the air in the alveoli of the lungs.**

The body is continually using oxygen and producing carbon dioxide and therefore the partial pressure of oxygen in the alveolar air (PA_{O_2}) and in the tissues will be lower than atmospheric air and the partial pressure of carbon dioxide (PA_{CO_2}) will be higher. The exact composition is a function of the composition of the inspired air, the rate of carbon dioxide production, and the ventilatory rate and volume. When breathing room air, the sum of the PA_{O_2} and PA_{CO_2} is fixed and any change results in an equal and opposite change in the other. A 10, 20, or 40 torr rise in PA_{CO_2} will result in a 10, 20, or 40 mm decrease in PA_{O_2}. The average PA_{CO_2} is 40 torr and the PA_{O_2} is 100 torr.

■ **Discuss the exchange of gases in the lungs and in the tissues.**

The exchange of gases in the lung through the alveolar membrane occurs by diffusion into the blood or in a reverse direction, depending upon the difference in the partial pressure of each gas on either side of the alveolar membrane. The diffusability of CO_2 is twenty times that of O_2. This fact helps explain a normal Pa_{CO_2} and a very low Pa_{CO_2} in some individuals with thickened alveolar membranes, as occurs in interstitial pneumonitis.

The normal exchange of oxygen and carbon dioxide in the lungs occurs as follows:

PA_{O_2} (alveolar air) = 100 torr
Pv_{O_2} (proximal alveolar capillary) = 40 torr

The 60 torr pressure gradient drives oxygen into the alveolar capillary blood from the alveoli.

PA_{CO_2} (alveolar air) = 40 torr
Pv_{CO_2} (proximal alveolar capillary) = 46 torr

The 6 torr pressure gradient and rapid diffusability of carbon dioxide drive it from the alveolar capillary blood into the alveoli.

Oxygen and carbon dioxide present in tissue capillary blood diffuse through the capillary membrane into the tissues or in a reverse direction depending upon the difference in pressure of the gas in question on either side of the membrane. The normal exchange of oxygen and carbon dioxide in the tissues occurs as follows:

Pa_{O_2} (proximal tissue capillary, arterial) $= 100$ torr
Po_2 tissue $= 30$ torr
Pv_{O_2} (distal tissue capillary, venous) $= 40$ torr

The 70 torr pressure gradient drives oxygen from the capillary blood into the tissue, from where it is returned to the lungs for re-oxygenation.

Pa_{CO_2} (proximal tissue capillary, arterial) $= 40$ torr
Pco_2 tissue $= 50$ torr
Pv_{CO_2} (distal tissue capillary, venous) $= 46$ torr

The 10 torr pressure gradient and rapid diffusability of carbon dioxide drive it from the tissue into the distal venous capillaries.

■ **Discuss the transportation of oxygen by blood.**

Oxygen is transported from the lungs to the tissue in the form of oxygen bound hemoglobin and oxygen dissolved in the plasma water. Only a small amount, 0.3 ml of oxygen per deciliter of blood, is carried in the dissolved state when atmospheric air is breathed. Each gram of hemoglobin when fully saturated with oxygen will combine with 1.34 ml of oxygen. Hemoglobin is nearly fully saturated with oxygen when the Po_2 is about 100 torr. The *oxygen capacity* of blood is defined as the amount of oxygen chemically combined with a deciliter of blood when the hemoglobin is fully saturated. It is readily calculated by multiplying the hemoglobin in grams per deciliter by 1.34. A person with a hemoglobin of 15 grams per deciliter will have an oxygen capacity of 20.1 ml per deciliter ($15 \times 1.34 = 20.1$). *Oxygen content* is the quantity of oxygen actually combined with hemoglobin.

The ratio of oxygen content to oxygen capacity times 100 is known as *percent oxygen saturation*. The percent saturation of hemoglobin is related to the Po_2. This relationship is readily understood if expressed graphically by plotting percent saturation on the ordinate and Po_2 on the abscissa. The curve obtained is called the *oxygen dissociation curve*. The curve is sigmoid in shape because the amount of oxygen bound to hemoglobin is not linearly related to the Po_2. As the Po_2 decreases, the percent saturation decreases slowly until the tension is about 50 to 55 torr, at which point oxygen is rapidly released from hemoglobin. This is important in that there must be a considerable reduction in the Po_2 of inspired air before any significant change in saturation occurs. As blood flows through the tissues which have a lower Po_2, oxygen is released until the Po_2 of the arterial blood approaches that of the tissue. Normally the Pa_{O_2} is reduced from 100 torr to 40 torr, which results in a release of one-third of the oxygen to the tissues. This provides a two-thirds reserve of oxygenated blood in the event that there is a reduction in oxygen in the inspired air.

■ **Discuss some factors which affect the dissociation of oxyhemoglobin.**

The configuration of the oxygen dissociation curve is described by the P_{50}. P_{50} is the P_{O_2} at which hemoglobin is 50% saturated. The normal P_{50} at a pH of 7.40 and a temperature of 37° C is about 27 torr. Several factors, namely, temperature, pH, P_{CO_2}, and the quantity of red cell 2,3-diphosphoglycerate (2,3-DPG), affect the dissociation of hemoglobin. An increase in P_{50} or a shift to the right of the oxygen dissociation curve indicates that the affinity of hemoglobin for oxygen is decreased and its ability to release oxygen to the tissues at a given P_{O_2} is increased. A decrease in P_{50} or a shift to the left of the oxygen dissociation curve indicates that the affinity of hemoglobin is increased and its ability to release oxygen to the tissues at a given P_{O_2} is decreased.

It has been long known that a decrease in pH, an increase in P_{CO_2}, and hyperthermia cause a shift to the right; whereas an increase in pH, a decrease in P_{CO_2}, and hypothermia result in a shift to the left of the oxygen dissociation curve. Recent studies have shown that, in addition to these factors, the position of the oxygen dissociation curve of adult hemoglobin is also affected by the interaction of hemoglobin with red cell organic phosphates. About 80% of the organic phosphates in the red cell is 2,3-DPG, a normal glycolytic intermediate of the Embden-Meyerhof cycle. ATP comprises most of the remainder of organic phosphate.

Red cell 2,3-DPG and the P_{50} are increased in clinical conditions in which there is an increase in oxygen demand or oxygen lack, such as in chronic lung disease, cyanotic heart disease, anemias secondary to iron deficiency, and red cell pyruvate kinase deficiency. It is also increased following vigorous exercise and adaptation to high altitudes.

Red cell 2,3-DPG and P_{50} are decreased following massive transfusion of stored blood and septic shock, in neonatal respiratory distress syndrome, and in carbon monoxide intoxication.

Persistent alkalosis or increased blood pH results in an increased production of red cell 2,3-DPG, whereas persistent acidosis or a decreased blood pH result in a decreased production of red cell 2,3-

DPG. These responses counteract the pH effect upon the oxygen dissociation curve.

■ **How are Po_2, percent O_2 saturation, and P_{50} measured?**

Po_2 is measured by a Clark electrode, which consists of a platinum cathode and an Ag/AgCl anode. The electrode is connected to an external low voltage power supply and is covered with a semipermeable membrane. The membrane permits oxygen to pass through to the cathode where the oxygen is reduced. An electrical current proportional to the Po_2 is generated.

The electrode is calibrated with humidified analyzed gas.

Percent oxygen saturation is now most commonly measured by one of several oximeters that are available. These oximeters determine spectrophotometrically the ratio of oxygenated hemoglobin to total hemoglobin present in a blood sample. The absorbance of the blood sample is measured at two specific wavelengths, one being the isosbestic point or the wavelength at which oxyhemoglobin and reduced hemoglobin have the same absorbance, and the other being at a wavelength in which oxyhemoglobin and reduced hemoglobin have different absorbances. The ratio of the absorbances at these two wavelengths is proportional to the percent oxygen saturation.

Percent saturation and Po_2 can be calculated also from an oxygen dissociation curve if the Po_2 or the percent saturation and the pH of the blood sample is known. This may be accurate if the P_{50} of the sample is within normal limits; however, when there is a shift to the right or left of the oxygen dissociation curve, the calculated parameter may be erroneous.

P_{50} is determined by measuring the Po_2, percent oxygen saturation, and pH on two aliquots of blood that have been equilibrated at 37° C in a tonometer with two gases of known oxygen content. The percent oxygen saturation of one aliquot should be slightly above 50% saturated and the other slightly below 50% saturated. The P_{50} can then be obtained by plotting the percent saturation against Po_2 corrected to pH 7.40. If a minicomputer is available it can be calculated using the Hill equation.

■ **Discuss the collection of blood for pH, Pco_2, and Po_2 studies.**

Venous blood, when properly drawn, is satisfactory for electrolytes, pH, and Pco_2 studies under almost all circumstances. Impressions gained from proper interpretation of the results obtained from venous blood will be the same as those obtained from arterial blood. Arterial blood studies are generally required when oxygen measurements are desired in addition to pH and Pco_2.

Medical technologists can and should be taught to obtain both venous and arterial blood so that electrolytes, pH, Pco_2, Po_2, and percent oxygen saturation determinations may be available at all times.

The collection of venous blood for acid-base studies should be done without prolonged venous stasis. The first blood obtained should be used for the determination of pH and Pco_2. If a tourniquet is used to locate a vein, it must not be released until after the blood is obtained or the pH will be falsely low.

Arterial blood can be readily obtained relatively painlessly without a tourniquet from the brachial, radial, or femoral arteries without the use of local anesthetic agents. After the needle is removed, firm pressure must be applied to the puncture site for 5 minutes.

Heparin is the only satisfactory anticoagulant for these determinations. Blood collection in heparinized glass or plastic syringes or vacuum tubes is satisfactory for only pH and Pco_2 studies. If Po_2 or percent oxygen saturation is desired, blood must be obtained anaerobically in heparinized tight-fitting syringes. Heparinized vacuum tubes are unsatisfactory for oxygen studies as they contain sufficient oxygen to substantially affect the Po_2 and percent oxygen saturation.

■ **Where is calcium located and what is its function?**

Ninety-nine percent of the body calcium is located in the bones and teeth. Most of the remaining 1% is located in the extracellular fluid. The normal serum calcium is 4.3 to 5.5 mEq/L. Fifty to 60% of serum calcium is ionized or complexed with citrate and other inorganic anions, with the remaining being bound to albumin and beta globulin. The ionized fraction is the physiologically important fraction.

Calcium is required to maintain bone and teeth development, neuromuscular function, and blood coagulation. It is also required for a variety of enzymatic reactions. Normal cellular membrane function and the maintenance of renal concentrating mechanisms also need this important cation.

■ **How do parathormone and thyrocalcitonin affect the serum calcium level?**

Parathormone (PTH) is a hormone secreted by the parathyroid glands. A reduced serum calcium level stimulates its release from the parathyroid glands. A high serum inorganic phosphorus, which may be present in chronic renal failure, results in lowering of serum calcium, which causes excessive secretion of PTH.

Parathormone stimulates an increased renal excretion of phosphate and a decreased excretion of calcium. It also promotes calcium absorption from the intestine and reabsorption of calcium and phosphate from the bones, resulting in an increased serum calcium.

Thyrocalcitonin is a hormone liberated by the parafollicular cells of the thyroid. It counteracts the actions of PTH in that bone reabsorption of calcium is inhibited and serum calcium is lowered. Its secretion is stimulated by an elevated serum calcium.

■ **Define hypercalcemia and list some of its causes. What other tests may be utilized to evaluate hypercalcemia?**

Hypercalcemia is a condition in which the serum calcium concentration is greater than 5.5 mEq/L.

Clinical conditions associated with hypercalcemia
1. Laboratory error
2. Neoplasia
   a. Metastatic to bone: lymphoma, leukemia, multiple myeloma, breast, lung, kidney, ovary, GI tract
   b. Primary tumors that produce PTH-like substances: hypernephroma, lung
3. Sarcoidosis
4. Hypervitaminosis D
5. Milk alkali syndrome
6. Hyperparathyroidism
7. Adrenal insufficiency
8. Idiopathic hypercalcemia of infancy
9. Acute skeletal atrophy of disuse
10. Hyperthyroidism

Laboratory tests to evaluate hypercalcemia
1. Repeat serum calcium
2. Serum inorganic phosphorus
3. Urinary calcium and phosphate excretion
4. Phosphate clearance test
5. Tubular reabsorption of phosphate
6. Alkaline phosphatase
7. Cortisone suppression test: 100-150 mg cortisone per day for 5-10 days results in lowering of serum calcium in most patients except those with primary hyperparathyroidism
8. Radioimmunoassay for PTH

■ **Define hypocalcemia and list some of its causes.**

Hypocalcemia is defined as a condition in which the serum calcium concentration is less than 4.5 mEq/L. The clinical sign of this condition is neuromuscular irritability (tetany).

Conditions associated with hypocalcemia
1. Laboratory error
2. Vitamin D deficiency—rickets, osteomalacia
3. Steatorrhea—sprue, pancreatic insufficiency
4. Tetany of newborn—secondary to high phosphate intake
5. Hypoparathyroidism—may be temporary following thyroidectomy
6. Pseudohypoparathyroidism—end organ refractoriness to PTH (Differentiated from true hypoparathyroidism by the Ellsworth-Howard test. The patient is given PTH and urinary phosphate excretion is measured. Phosphate excretion is increased in hypoparathyroidism but not in pseudohypoparathyroidism.)
7. Renal failure with hyperphosphatemia
8. Pancreatitis, acute
9. Pregnancy with poor intake of calcium

■ **What is the distribution of magnesium and what is its function?**

Magnesium is the fourth most abundant extracellular cation and the second most abundant intracellular cation. Seventy percent of the body magnesium is complexed with calcium and phosphorus in the bones. Thirty-five percent of the plasma magnesium is protein bound. Magnesium is the only cation in the cerebrospinal fluid that has a higher concentration than in the plasma. The normal serum magnesium is 1.5 to 2.5 mEq/L.

Magnesium is an activator for many enzyme systems involved in the metabolism of carbohydrates and protein. Magnesium, as calcium, affects neuromuscular irritability.

Magnesium is absorbed by the small intestine. Renal excretion is inhibited by parathormone. A low serum magnesium stimulates the parathyroid to release PTH.

■ **Discuss hypomagnesemia.**

Hypomagnesia is a condition in which the serum magnesium is less than 1.5 mEq/L. Magnesium deficiency states occur when there is a deficient intake, when there is poor absorption by the small bowel, or when there is excessive loss from the urinary or gastrointestinal tract. Endocrinologic disorders may also be a cause.

Symptoms may include tetany, seizures, hyperexcitability, and psychotic behavior. Hypomagnesemia may coexist with hypocalcemia or with normocalcemic states. Tetany with hypomagnesemia but normal serum calcium and pH has been recognized as the "magnesium deficiency tetany syndrome." The difference between hypocalcemic and hypomagnesemic tetany is determined by measurements of the serum content of these cations.

Hypomagnesemia has been associated with the following disorders: various malabsorption syndromes, alcoholism, both hyper- and hypoparathyroidism, diabetic ketoacidosis, chronic renal disease of various etiologies, burns, diuretic therapy, pancreatitis, and tumors metastatic to bone.

■ **Define hypermagnesemia.**

Hypermagnesemia is a condition in which the serum magnesium is greater than 2.5 mEq/L. Hypermagnesemia is most often seen in renal failure or is iatrogenic in nature. It has also been reported in diabetic coma and in patients with megacolon. Coma occurs with magnesium levels above 14 mEq/L.

Index

t indicates reference to table.